Sparks Start Fires
A Guide for Dreamers Who Are Also Doctors

Julie K. Gunther, M.D, FAAFP
Owner, sparkMD, LLC
Family Physician

To my colleagues, because we must.
And to our patients, because we will.

Truth is like fire;
to tell the truth is to glow and burn.

-Gustav Klimt

Table of Contents

Table of Contents

When old age shall this generation waste,
Thou shalt remain, in midst of other woe
Than ours, a friend to man, to whom thou
say'st,

"Beauty is truth, truth beauty,—that is all
Ye know on earth, and all ye need to know."

-John Keats, *Ode On a Grecian Urn*

I've always been a builder, tinkerer and a serial hobbyist. As soon as I come close, or feel close to mastery of a thing, I move on. Family medicine and, now, direct primary care, have been the perfect fit for my ever-curious, ever-distracted interests in all things people, buildings, art and business.

I love solving problems. Geometry was a turning point for me in high school. Once my brain grasped the concept of thinking about proofs, my whole world changed. If we can't do a thing the way we do it, can we do it backwards? What is the hack? How can we deliver on the spirit of a thing…but even better?

In college, my world opened to notions of social responsibility. Ingrained was the idea that when we are present, we are participants. Whether we put our heads in the sand, raise our hands in defiance, stay quiet or protest loudly, all are a choice and a form of participation. So long as we work in a place and with a people, we represent that place, their rules, their system and their ways. Even if we don't agree with them.

In healthcare, independence is an act of defiance.

This is my story of how I became a direct primary care physician. Here are the seeds that were sewn when I worked in the system and how those seeds grew. It is my hope that by telling my story of becoming the physician I set out to be, I can empower physician colleagues to find the heart of their work again.

There are many personal and patient stories that illustrate not only how broken our healthcare system is, but how much hope and compassion remain shared in the therapeutic space between provider and patient, no matter how much anyone tries to digitize it.

We are not widgets.

The provision of care cannot be done in an assembly line.

This is the beauty of what we do... the beauty of doctoring. The only way to doctor, is to remove every last ounce of anything unnecessary, extraneous or distracting from the relationship between physician and patient. The compassion, humanity and shared experience that exists between a person needing help and the person working to provide it is the heart of medicine. And this heart exists in the intangible, unquantifiable in-between.

Dr. Julie Gunther, M.D., FAAFP
4.2020

If I know what love is . . .
It is because of you.

-Herman Hesse

In 2009, at the age of 34, I became a full-fledged Board Certified family physician. My husband and I moved back to Idaho with our one and four year old daughters. We'd missed the mountains, the outdoor lifestyle, Subarus, 'hippie food' and all things Northwest. We were looking forward to life being different after ten rigorous years of postgraduate education, medical school and residency.

The days in residency are long.

The years are longer.

Those three years felt, and still feel, like a lifetime.

I wanted to be a 'do everything' doctor. I trained to deliver babies, cast fractures, remove skin cancers and so much more. I was excited to be the Swiss Army knife of medicine, which was always my vision of doctoring. Shortly before residency ended, I spent six weeks working in a rural mountain town in Central Idaho, with a population of 3,400, give or take seasonal workers. I had spent much of my childhood there picking mushrooms and huckleberries in the woods and swimming in the large mountain lake. Living and working in McCall, Idaho, was beyond the summation of my dream.

The doctors in McCall were and are mostly primary care physicians. In six weeks, I cared for patients in motor vehicle collisions, critically ill elderly people, and a young woman in a cardiac arrhythmia from methamphetamine and caffeine use. I delivered babies, amputated and repaired a rancher's middle finger and learned about acupuncture. Rural family physicians are the obstetricians, the surgeons, the trauma doctors, the critical care physicians, the subspecialists, the ER doctors, the paediatricians. Rural family doctors, well-trained, have a profound capacity for comprehensive care.

I *loved* everything about this.

I was rarely home. People recognized me at the grocery store where I did quick "urgent care" consults. The pharmacist recognized me by voice. When the phone rang at the cabin in the middle of the night my husband got up to feed our one year old and I drove into town to see a patient in the ER. One of my attendings, a senior physician who had worked in McCall for decades, lamented how he avoided town because he needed a break from the community. But I felt so alive. It was everything I wanted for myself.

But it wasn't something that would work for the part of my life that most sustained me. My family.

The process of becoming a fully-trained family physician was exhausting not only for me but also for my husband. While I gained weight, had a premature delivery, lost my hair, ignored what was later found to be a breast cancer, I was also so excited as I worked to be the doctor I envisioned I would be.

My amazing, rational, supportive, funny and infinitely loving husband's time while I worked in McCall was another step down the never-ending rabbit hole of me being ever-absent. After nine years of going to bed alone, cooking meals that got cold before I ate them, paying the bills, finishing dates after I'd returned to the hospital and raising kids with a partially-there partner, he had run out of steam. This all-in rural family physician job offered him no light at the end of the residency tunnel. He was losing hope that we were going to cultivate anything close to the life we had envisioned together.

One afternoon near the end of my rotation we were about to go look at a ranch home on 40 acres. I was bubbling over with excitement. He asked me:

"Julie, can you be *a* doctor? . . .

or do you have to be *the* doctor?

Because if you have to be *the* doctor, I don't know if I can do this anymore.

But if you can be *a* doctor, I can support that."

This is no place for a girl on fire.

-Susanne Collins, *Catching Fire*

In late 2009 we bought a home in Boise, Idaho, settled down, learned all about Montessori education for our girls and got on with life. I took a four-day-a-week job as an employed outpatient family physician with the local hospital system. I went back to the gym and started meal planning. I lost fifty pounds. We began building a life with me being *a* doctor. And for a while, things worked.

As our lives were evolving so was the healthcare system. Family physicians in cities were rarely, if ever, doing hospital work or obstetrics anymore. I stopped doing OB, ER, trauma and inpatient work, each of which represented a tremendously important part of the full patient care continuum. I missed all of it.

For about two years, I built my practice and reputation as an employed physician. In that short time, I gained and lost a partner, gained and lost another partner, had three different office managers and had the physical location of my practice moved once. I volunteered to launch an on-site employer clinic where my medical assistant and I worked once weekly. I didn't know it then, but that on-site clinic was the teeniest of DPC seeds.

Just before Christmas of 2011, my newish physician colleague was in the middle of a breakdown related to depression, lost idealism and giving too much of herself. She had been in and out of clinic and I had been covering patient care so she could get caught up on notes. It wasn't working. I was looking forward to a week off when she informed me she was unable to cover the clinic over the holiday. Simultaneously, my medical assistant let me know, through a lot of tears, that she was going to work with the new internal medicine physician who had been added to our office. She was afraid they were going to shutter the family medicine portion of the practice and move me across town. With her young girls and role at home, she wasn't in a position to work at a different clinic.

In my experience, it takes about three years to build glorious, correct, comprehensive patient charts. Three years, strangely, also seems to be the EMR lifespan- or at least it was earlier in my career. Over Christmas of 2011, plans were laid to convert all of the physician charts from a program called 'ecw' to 'Epic'. In the span of one day, I was looking at going down to a one provider practice, restarting with a new medical assistant and having to figure out how to re-build 3000+ patient charts while learning a new EMR. On top of this was that I was RVU contracted with no accommodation or acknowledgement of the uncompensated administrative lift that would need to be done, again, to rebuild my practice.

I was done.

I realized that I had accepted being *a* doctor, being employed, with the notion that doing so provided benefits I couldn't provide for myself. Stability. Income. Clean rooms. Staffing. Medical records. A supply chain. Shared responsibility. "Off time" because there was a *team*. All of the sudden, though, through a haze of anger and fatigue I realized the system offered me nothing. No guarantees. A revolving door of staff who didn't answer to me. Inconsistent supply chains. Unstocked rooms. And no pens. (for real!).

My Medicare primary care incentive dollars- that I earned- were garnished by the system. When I asked questions about the piece of paper that was placed on my desk more than a year after the Medicare incentive dollars were paid, which stated I consented to my employer claiming these dollars I was told I could "sign the page or find a new job". My three years of charting were rendered irrelevant, with debate that the best option for re-entering of charts was for physicians to do it themselves over weekends and afterhours. My working relationship with my amazing medical assistant was so efficient we grossly exceeded all RVU's. Even that wasn't valued enough to provide her or I with the resources we needed to manage our patient panel. Often if she or I didn't handle something ourselves, it didn't get handled. So we both worked, late into the evening and weekends, at times, to make sure everything was handled.

Stability, income, benefits, staffing, medical records (EMR), boundaries, supply chain, partnerships, shared responsibility, pens, functional bathrooms...

All a no.

The system wasn't handling anything consistently, or in a way that made it easier to provide seamless patient care.

After my MA told me she was switching doctors, I called the senior physician who coordinated the call group I was in. I informed him that I wanted a transfer to the family medicine clinic around the corner from my house- or I would be quitting effective immediately. I left, drove the half hour home, walked in past my family and my in-laws visiting for the holidays, went straight upstairs to my bed, and cried.

The next morning the physician in charge of the family medicine division called to ask about my partner and about coverage over the holidays. I frankly don't remember what I said except it involved something along the lines of: "I am taking ten days off, I am unavailable to all further conversation, it is your job to figure out how to cover our clinic needs and I will not be answering or having any further discussions until I am back." He had always been very good to me and I had never spoken to him in that way. But I hung up and took my kids to their swimming lesson. For the first time since starting medical school, I earnestly turned off my phone for 10 full days.

The strange thing is, even now, everyone except my medical assistant seemed surprised at my anger, my need for time off, and my request for transfer.

How hard do you bend something before it breaks?

A month or so later my MA, my physician partner, a few administrators, the clinic manager and I had a meeting to coordinate my clinic transfer. My partner believed I had been plotting the departure for some time and was livid. In her year or so with the system, nothing ever happened quickly. She stopped speaking to me, locked herself in her exam rooms to do administrative work and our relationship deteriorated.

My partner's nurse asked to transfer with me. While I declined, the administrator in charge of physician services informed me I couldn't deny a qualified applicant.

The administrator who had made innumerable unkept commitments to me and both of my physician partners, who was the force behind mandating that physicians should do their own EMR chart re-entry, who asked us to move from our first clinic then coordinated the movement of internal medicine physicians into our second clinic, and the administrator who refused to provide more staffing resources walked out of the meeting with me.

When we were sufficiently out of ear shot of the other participants, she leaned over and whispered to me, "I always wanted you at that other clinic."

After my move in 2012, I stopped tolerating dysfunction.

I just couldn't do it anymore. Not that I became some sort of fearless empowered crusader-that took some time. But I stopped being so soft. In doing so, I almost lost my job once, got called a "bitch" behind my back and I made a lot more work for myself and everyone around me.

Something in medicine began changing then, too. Balls were getting dropped on patient care all over the place. Despite using six sigma and lean and automotive factory models of systematization, the actual delivery of care-- meaning meeting a person's needs when they had them and following through to make sure a proper outcome occurred- the health care system as a whole started to fall on its face. Patients were sent from my primary care clinic to the ER for critical issues and then sent home only to return the next day. Patients were being discharged from the hospital before they were stable and following up in the primary care clinic (if they could get in), very ill, only to be sent to the ER then back home. Around and around we all went. My practice's wait times for new patients exceeded 3 months. Families regularly told me they were sent to the urgent care by my front desk staff because I had no openings. In my five years as an employed outpatient physician within this system I twice, as in on two distinct occasions, declined add on patients. But daily, people told me they were told I had no openings. Friends with personal texts from me saying, "yes, come in and we can do a quick visit" were turned away at the front desk. One by one patient stories lined up...and then fell apart.

With each domino, I gained more clarity about why I morally could not call myself a doctor and remain in the system. One by one I collected examples of why I could no longer consent to be a part of something so broken..

Why did I have to leave the system? Why did I have to open my own clinic? Why did I have to stop taking insurance payments? Why did I have to do things differently?

Because I still wanted to be a doctor.

Morally, I could no longer uphold a construct that was harming people at a faster and faster pace. My name was on the front door but I had zero control over anything that happened in the building, including patient care.

I felt like I was on-fire, daily. Sometimes it a fire of inspiration, a passion for how things *should* be. I knew what caring for people should look like. I was seeing that I could care for people without the system and to believe I could do so in a way that had more integrity, more consistency and more transparency. I could see a path of care where I could keep my word and be the doctor I set out to be. These were the good days. Or hours. At other times the fire was just straight rage. Stuff it down, hold it in, don't say anything irrevocable rage. Rage over the harm being done in so many small and large and repeated ways over and over and over again in the name of health care.

I began to realize if I didn't get out, I was going to burn things down.

This is the way the world ends
This is the way the world ends
This is the way the world ends
Not with a bang but with a whimper.

~TS. Eliot The Hollow Men

Steven was my last domino.

Even years later, it's very difficult to write about Steven*. I think about him every day. I wish things had been different.

Steven was sixty-eight when I met him. For the sake of privacy, just in case, his name wasn't really Steven. A few of the details of his story are changed, or muted by my memory, but the spirit of Steven, and what happened to him, is retained.

Steven was a big-bellied, yellow-tinged, bearded grandpa-type, who despised being vulnerable. He was depressed in the way that men who used to ride Harleys are depressed, gruff and reluctant with a penchant for sarcasm and short phrases. He did not like going to the doctor. If his body hadn't let him down, I don't think we would have met. (All of that is true about Steven).

Steven's chief complaint at his first visit was shortness of breath. I remember talking to him and typing while he sat across from me and thinking he seemed like an overall ok kind of guy. No history of COPD, no history of smoking, dyspnea was probably just obesity. Easy peasy. When Steven stood up to walk three feet to sit on the exam table he could barely breathe. He was catastrophically ill but didn't want me to see it and didn't want to deal with it.

That moment has stuck with me. I met Steven in late 2011, before my practice fell apart and I switched clinics. I was growing in my clinical confidence and still naïve about the brokenness of the healthcare system. In our first visit, I had made my assessment of things before Steven stood up. For a moment I was feeling pretty capable.

The contrast between his health story and his symptoms with minimal exertion was remarkable. I had jumped to conclusions to get through my allotted ten minute visit. Ready to be done and move on to the next patient, I realized I was being hasty and judgemental. I was moving too fast to provide the care I believed everyone deserved. I wasn't paying attention to Steven. The algorithms, and notes and check boxes were done, though.

What if I had acted on my first assumptions? Steven's self-report contrasted so dramatically with what I saw when he had to do a minimal task. My lesson in that moment was to slow down and do the job of caring properly. Every time. Use all the tools- patient information, vital signs, physical exam, critical thinking- even when things seem obvious. A person may report what they want but the body carries the story.

My second lesson in that moment with Steven was that most people, most of the time, do not want to see a doctor. When people cross the threshold into the exam room they are doing so because they believe something is wrong. In every single encounter people deserve a pause. They deserve our attention. And they deserve the dignity and respect of time and an earnest assessment.

I took care of Steven for the next four years. He followed me when I moved across town. He eventually opened up a little bit and would talk about his frustration with not being what he once was. He tried to lose weight and improve his self-care. But life got messy. In spite of long counseling-like visits (which always put me way behind with my clinic schedule but that just was what it was then), encouragement of mental health services, debates about antidepressants, spirituality and working on correcting past wrongs, Steven just couldn't get traction. He lost his house and generally got older, heavier and more depressed.

And then he just couldn't do it anymore.

Steven came into clinic one day and asked if I thought he should have bariatric surgery. We had a long discussion. I didn't feel he was ready but believed that it was perhaps his last shot at radical personal transformation. He was exhausted with life and the weight of it all. He went to the after-hours seminar, signed up, and had surgery.

For about six months, things went well. He dropped a remarkable amount of weight, could breathe, could sleep and could care for himself again. He moved out of the trailer in his son's backyard and got a town house. He bought himself a new Ford F-250. He told me how he loved driving his grandson around in it. Life was getting better. His labs were normal, he was more ambulatory, his mood improved and, while he was grossly noncompliant with the post-bariatric surgery diet recommendations, things were going in the right direction.

I came into clinic one day to a series of messages that Steven had been vomiting all weekend. He did confess he was eating chicken wings and maybe swallowed a few bones. We reviewed the bariatric surgery compliant foods and I had him follow up a day or so later.

He was still nauseated and cyclically vomiting.

I started to see Steven weekly. At first his labs were normal, his vitals were normal and everything seemed circumstantial to his bariatric surgery. He had a tough time getting follow-up with his surgeon and, when he did, they felt nothing was related to his surgery and sent him back to me. Intermittently, his liver numbers were mildly elevated and we worked this up without findings. With his history of obesity and recent massive weight loss this wasn't all that unusual. When they persisted, I sent him to gastroenterology. They felt his findings were consistent with fatty liver and sent him back to me, as well.

Steven kept coming in and things just kept getting worse.

He lost control of his bowels in his new F-250, which was a source of great shame and something he only shared with me because he refused to come in for a follow up visit. When I asked him why, it was because he couldn't maintain continence for the twenty minute drive.

So I did home visits.

Eventually, Steven became dehydrated and couldn't be cared for at home. So I referred him to the ER.

And they gave him fluids and sent him home to follow up with me.

So I called gastroenterology. And they declined the referral feeling they had nothing further to offer.

And he declined at home, so I sent him to the ER. He went; and they sent him home.

And around and around we went.

I think once or twice he did get admitted, eventually, for a day or two. I know he stayed overnight once after I called and pled with the ER doctor to keep him. But every time, he came back to the outpatient setting to see me in 'follow up'. And every time he was a little bit worse.

Steven's final outpatient visit was one of the last visits I did before I gave notice that I was quitting my system job. He had been discharged from the hospital two days prior and came in with his son, which was unusual. Generally he came in alone. That day, he looked terrible. He was dishevelled and his loose skin hung from his cheeks. He couldn't lift his head up. His muscles just wouldn't do it.

With his chin on his chest and his eyes looking downward, I asked Steven if he was able to lift his head two days prior when he left the hospital. His answer was, "sort of".

I did the best I could but again, I told Steven he needed to go to the hospital. I asked his son to take him to the ER and to leave him there.

After clinic I went to the hospital, found Steven and waited in his room with him until the hospitalist on duty presented to complete his admission.

The hospitalist on duty was one of my medical school colleagues. One of the best doctors I'd ever met. We studied next to each other. When I quit, went home, went on a walk…she kept studying. She'd never stop. Not to eat, not to walk, just kept learning and learning and learning so she could be good enough.

I told her all about Steven. Steven in the real world. Steven outside of the hospital. Steven in his F-250. Steven the Grandpa. I told her that I wanted her to be his hospitalist. No one else. No transfers, no early discharges. I told her that he was not to be discharged until they called me. I would be seeing him daily; social rounds to coordinate care, check on him and see if we could make some progress. I asked her to agree with me that he needed to be stable more than 24 hours before he was sent home.

I begged, please, please, help me figure out what is wrong with Steven.

That time they kept him.

During that hospitalization, Steven would start to get better and his hospitalist team would discuss discharge. They'd call me and say, "we're going to discharge him". Three times I said: "how about one more day?" and he would go down-hill again.

One day while in the hospital checking on Steven I crossed paths with a palliative care physician. He had been asked to consult on Steven's case. I asked if we could re-engage gastroenterology. Steven's liver numbers had been waxing and waning, in a way that just didn't make any sense. I had wondered for months (and asked intermittently) about the utility of a liver biopsy. For what reason? I really didn't fully know. Imaging was unrevealing earlier in the course of his issues. And his labs varied with his diet, hydration status and overall well being, or lack thereof.

Because Steven's overall trajectory was poor, the inpatient team, the palliative care doctor and even the gastroenterologist pushed back- what would a liver biopsy change? There was no overt evidence this was cirrhosis and no mass lesions.

Eventually, however, a liver biopsy was done. Steven had infiltrative hepatocellular carcinoma.

Steven went home to his son's. I remained his doctor but this time, in my role as an Associate Hospice Medical director. For a few months his nausea, vomiting and diarrhea were better. He spent time with his grandkids. He reconnected with his son. I like to think he had a few good days.

One of my last conversations with Steven was a week before his birthday. His son had secretly bought tickets for them both to go to his favorite college football team's homecoming game.

Steven passed away a few days before making the trip.

Steven's care haunts me. I think it's because the circumstances around his care were so broken that I am ashamed. I can try to be objective and feel like I did everything I rightfully could do. Home visits. Hospital visits. Advocating at the bedside. Repeated calls to the ER, to consulting physicians, coaching the family. But the truth is what happened to Steven makes me ashamed to be a doctor. It makes me ashamed to have had *anything* to do with the healthcare system. His care in the last year of his life affirmed all of the negative things said about our health care system and about health care providers.

The last year of Steven's life and the events around it robbed him of his dignity. The system, which I was a part of, did not deliver on *anything* we inherently committed to do. And it robbed him of time. The last months of his life were spent in discomfort, traveling from home to hospital to home to clinic with uncertainty, escalating medical bills, minimal answers and limited compassion.

It is because of Steven that I had to leave the system.

And it is because of Steven that I will *never* ever work for anyone but my patients ever again.

You never change things by fighting
the existing reality. To change something,
build a new model that makes the existing
model obsolete.

-Buckminster Fuller

Start your own direct primary care practice because it will save you to be the doctor you always wanted to be.

I am a woman of many hats. Mother, entrepreneur, small business owner, physician, friend, dabbling photographer, closet seamstress, wife, occasional blogger, art teacher, hospice director, advocate.... many many hats. But I am not an accountant, a lawyer, an insurance agent, nor the only passionate direct primary care physician. That is my caveat.

This book is borne of the desire to start from the very beginning to answer the question: How do I leave the system, stop doing what I know how to do the only way I know how to do it and liberate myself to be the doctor I wanted to be in the first place? This is one way. There are A LOT of different ways to do this.

Hopefully this will provide pearls and some basic guideposts so you know that the journey to independence is not only possible but enjoyable. Nothing takes the place of your own vision, your own clear passion as to how to make your community and your role within your community, better. Nothing takes the place of your own unique, thoughtful solutions, empowered with vision.

Do what you know you can do. What you know your community needs. Live the vision you had when you decided to become a physician in the first place. Your world, and the world of those for whom you care, will be transformed because of it.

Health Insurance is not health care. And, either way, it's all broken.

When I was building my confidence to start our small medical clinic there were so many steps. One was to get an LLC, S-Corp, pLLC and I had no clue how to do this.

Frankly, I was overwhelmed.

And then I drove by a taco stand.

In a more agricultural part near where I live, on the side of the road was a revised shed turned into a taco shack with a proud, homemade sign that said, "Tony's Tacos, LLC."

And hit me. We can get so rigid with what is familiar. The process of becoming a physician is rigorous and demands daily learning. It is work. It is constant dives until the uncertain. It is learning from others, from books, from articles, from videos, from patients. All. Day. Long. Business is no different.

In business we use the phrase 'pivot'. Changing rotations every 4-6 weeks for more than five years is the consummate exercise in 'pivoting'. Doctors know how to work. We know how to learn. We know how to pivot. We know hussle. If Tony can form an LLC, you can too.

Starting your own business requires curiosity, the desire to solve problems, the ability to pivot and work. And we know how to do all of those things.

If you've made it this far you're interested in doing something different. And, I suspect, you already know how broken our healthcare system is.

Health insurance is not health CARE. Period. Just like car insurance isn't Danika Patrick driving a race car. Somewhere, someone, somehow, thought a plastic card with a code number from some people in suits in a big city equated to compensated care. And somehow we all signed up to agree to this. But we don't have to.

The practice of medicine has become virtually unsustainable. We feel it every day. Family physicians are the most highly paid administrative assistants our country has. (Actually, I take that back. Corporate administrative assistants make more than family docs.) Anyway, in case you are a dictation goddess or by some amazing cosmic event have a scribe at your beck and call, you know it is not unusual for a physician, a PhD equivalent, to perform data entry tasks upwards of 4-6 hours daily, now estimated to be at least 40% of the total work day.

So, here's why it stinks to be a primary care physician in our present health care construct:

1. Suicide
2. Deferred income
3. Shit rolls down hill
4. No one answers their phone anymore
5. On a W2 you get NO WHERE with taxes
6. Abusive, or, at best, unresponsive administration
7. The faster you run, the farther behind you get

8. Loss of autonomy

9. Apologizing

10. Insufficient time to do quality work

11. Loss of role as patient advocate

I suspect you could articulate many more of your own deeply personal reasons for why what you are doing now, and how you are doing it, no longer fits with your own vision for providing the best care. With all of these challenges, are you still the doctor you set out to be?

Do you remember your personal statement or your medical school interview? Maybe that conversation you had where you convinced your parents/partner/anyone, really, that you were going to be a doctor? What did you tell people, back in the day when you were all naive and inspired?

And what are you now?

How much of what you are now is NOTHING like what you want to be? What would doctoring look like of you could eliminate all of that. What if you could get rid of 90% of the things that are a waste of your inspiration, that kill your idealism, that make your bone marrow hurt...what if you designed a working construct that eliminated all, or at least most, of *that?*

In 6-9 months, you have the opportunity for that version of you and your work life to be gone.

I promise.

A former president of the American Academy of Family Physicians at a conference I went to in 2014 noted, "we [family physicians] have to stop rolling over and showing our soft pink underbelly". We under-code, we under-bill, we over-provide and, in doing so, we wear ourselves out. We are leaving this profession early and in droves. We deter our younger colleagues, our kids, and the motivated capable young neighbor from a life in medicine. Why? Because it is terrible. And we know it.

But it doesn't have to be.

There are a lot of professional ways to articulate why we leave medicine: "the present practice environment is unsustainable". "My present patient outcomes are such that I have converted to an urgent care model to accommodate the local primary care shortage". Call it what you want, phrase it as you will, but let's be honest. Family medicine (or internal medicine, or, really, all of primary care) for people who were interested in the service part in the first place, distils down to absolutely nothing when you remove the opportunity for shared experiences and for service. What we're left with is churn-and-burn, administrative abuse and a job that as my last shadowing medical student (before I left the system) stated: "is totally sucky".

Our training comes at tremendous personal and social cost. So having physicians who are disengaged, depressed, suicidal and wanting to leave medicine is a tremendous tragedy and growing social problem.

T he name "Dr. Marcus Welby" comes up not infrequently in my present circles as the iconoclastic representation of what doctors used to be. *Marcus Welby, M.D.* was a kindly family TV doctor who did house calls and knew most of his patients by first name. We make TV shows about things that capture our imagination--about things that interest us. *Marcus Welby, M.D.* ran for seven years and inspired many young people to a career in primary care.

In a post on KevinMD, retired physician Dr. Rosenberg argued that the Marcus Welby ideal "has gone the way of the horse and buggy". I disagree. I've never watched *Marcus Welby, MD*. But I was inspired by the idea of a small town country doctor. I was not inspired to be a physician with the vision that at five o'clock I would fall back into the fold of my community and not contribute. I didn't apply to medical school because I, one day, wanted to have a 'day job as a doctor'. I wanted to be a physician. I wanted to be *the* physician.

There are just some professions for which who you are and what you do are very intimately intertwined.

It's time to live your vision.

Go back to that page where you wrote down what you set out to be. Still can't remember? Call your mom. Or ask your spouse. What were you when you envisioned your best you?

While this all sounds hokey-- here's my answer...maybe it will help. I wanted to buy an old barn. A big old barn.

I wanted to gut it, live in the upstairs, big roughhewn beams, energy inefficiency and all, and I wanted the ground floor to be part community center, part 24/7 medical clinic. I wanted to drive a 4-wheeler around in the middle of the night delivering babies (I am not a fan of horses). This cinematic vision was rooted in one ideal. I wanted to use my abilities to help people. To counsel. To welcome. To make a difference. To be a consistent, capable, honest, kind resource for my community. To give of my time and the privilege of my education to help people stay on track, get on track and make their own lives better.

Mr. Rogers said, "always look for the helpers". In spite of all of the Michaela Quinn Medicine Woman Disney thematics in my original vision there was one completely authentic core value. I wanted to build something. Something better than myself. Better than what a place, and a people, started with.

You can't build a damn thing when your hands are tied, your vision squelched, your resources sparse and your voice hushed. You just can't. No matter how capable you once were.

You have choices.

So, now that I've hopefully provided you with enough evidence that I wanted to be the family doctor of lore, explained all of my professional woes and limitations, here's where things get fun.

You don't have to leave medicine.

You don't have to stop being a doctor.

You don't have to sit across the table from people who lecture you about 'patient care' who have never even taken care of one patient.

You don't have to stop believing in your original, authentic vision for being the doctor you want to be.

Get your vision back and move forward.

W hen you've decided that yes, you love being a
doctor and, yes, if you could be the doctor you set out to
be this would all be worth it then you're ready to move
forward.

And, here's what's going to happen:

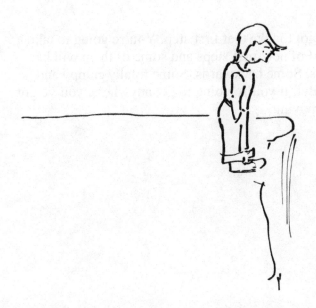

You're there. Now what? Everything is new. Everything
is foreign. And, all of the sudden, every next step is inter-
related.

Here's what you have to do:

Jump.

Yup.

Jump.

(No, don't jump for real but, metaphorically.....)

Jump.

You've got to take that first step. You're going to take a whole lot of new first steps and some of them will be sideways. Some backwards. Some totally crappy and wrong. But, if you're going to get anywhere, you've got to start moving.

Getting from Here to Freedom in 20 Steps

If you despise reading or just read way too much UpToDate to consider reading recreationally, I get it. The following seven pages have a list. This is how you start a DPC practice (or, probably any small business, for the most part). This is certainly not the only check list out there and not necessarily comprehensive for every kind of direct primary care practice. But it is a guide.

The remainder of this book is designed to walk through these start-up steps to help you march through this check-list and open your own, independent practice. Resources, how we did it, considerations and 'hacks" are delivered to help you get from 'what am I doing" to open as quickly as possible in twenty steps.

It will help you with the remainder of this book, with your business plan and you can *always* scratch out your answers and revise.

Here we GO!

DPC Start-Up Timeline

You're Inspired: What Next?
-more than 6 months prior to opening-

☐ Define your Vision
☐ Think BIG: What do you want to do with your life? Can you SEE it? Do you still want to be a doctor? (are you sure?)
☐ Where do you want your practice to be?
☐ Do you want a partner/a mid level?
☐ Do you want to do inpatient? OB? Home visits?
☐ Are there other particular circumstances specific to your dream practice?

Budget

☐ Understand your home budget.
☐ Do 3 months cash for all elective spending
☐ Figure out how much you need to earn for the next 1,2,3 years.
☐ Get money back: sell, quit, add, modify
☐ Do you need a side job?

Get Educated

☐ www.dpcfrontier.com
☐ www.dpcalliance.org
☐ www.dpcare.org
☐ www.atlas.md
☐ google!
☐ Hint Community Forum
☐ Research YOUR state laws around cash-based and retainer-based practices

Brainstorm

- Carry a notebook for ideas
- Get a business credit card
- Start a pinterest page
- Start saving documents in one place (gsuites, evernote, dropbox)
- You might as well splurge on an ipad now (save the receipt!)

Know What You've Got
-6 months out-

- Review your existing contracts and consider what needs negotiated
- How many patients do you have now?
- How far are you moving?
- How much can you communicate?
- Can you solicit patients before you leave/quit/move?
- Maintain a list of patients you would like to have in your new practice.
- Who is your "ideal" customer/patient?

Money, Money, Money

- Where can you get money?
- How much money does your vision need?

Build your Team

- Find a mentor (dpcalliance.org and/or dpcfrontier.com)
- SCORE, SBA, BNI, local college/university
- Visit your mentors by phone, email, in person.

- [ ] Talk/email DPC docs who you feel you have similar philosophy to- pick their brains
- [ ] Interview business accountants
- [ ] Interview commercial real estate agents
- [ ] Interview small business lawyers
- [ ] Get a BUSINESS banker
- [ ] Go to DPC conferences

Location, Location, Location
-5 months out-

- [ ] Find a location. Start up vs. long term
- [ ] Lease vs. buy
- [ ] Ask for 3-6 mos FREE
- [ ] Ask for landlord to pay for build-out
- [ ] Look around for retiring/retired physicians/dentists for leasable space

Start Acting like a DPC Doctor NOW

Act Like a Pro

- [ ] Get a professional photograph taken.
- [ ] Update/create a Linked IN profile
- [ ] Create a business Facebook page, Instagram & Twitter. **Try to use/get the same handle**
- [ ] Mind your on-line reputation.

Build Your Brand

- [ ] Decide on your business model
- [ ] Decide on your model: membership + visit fee? Membership with visit limits, Membership with incidentals charged at cost plus? Membership

with most included except some incidentals?
Membership plus insurance billing? Your call
- ☐ Decide on your NAME.
- ☐ Buy your URL
- ☐ Get a logo

Lay the Corner Stones

- ☐ Decide on your transition plan
- ☐ Decide on your financing: benefactor, venture capitol, savings, side jobs, loans, bonus, SBA?
- ☐ Get your LLC, S-Corp or pLLC
- ☐ Get a phone number
- ☐ Get a basic flash page where people can provide their info to get more of YOUR info
- ☐ Get a basic business card

The Nuts & Bolts

- ☐ Decide on your pricing
- ☐ Decide on your patient volume
- ☐ Decide on your offerings
- ☐ Decide on labs, imaging, meds (yay or nay) and pricing model (cost + 10%), Cost plus "fill/draw fee" etc...
- ☐ Try out EMRs.
- ☐ Write a Business Plan.
- ☐ Plan Your Transition
- ☐ Review your existing contracts and consider what needs negotiated.
- ☐ Think ahead to health, disability and life insurance (while you can access HR)
- ☐ Consider CME to augment your DPC offerings (procedures etc).
- ☐ Plan for townhalls if you can.
- ☐ Give notice in writing!

Bricks & Mortar
-4 months to open-

- ☐ Don't forget about zoning considerations
- ☐ Apply for licenses/permitting/look at OSHA rules
- ☐ Arrange/make sure insurance contracts are terminated
- ☐ Be mindful of address changes needed
- ☐ Mind your google/online address/info/reputation

Network
-3 months out-

- ☐ Master your elevator speech
- ☐ Join your local chamber of commerce
- ☐ Join a local BNI chapter
- ☐ Get a storage unit/POD/make room in your garage unless you have early access to your space
- ☐ Decide on overall clinic aesthetic/design and begin purchasing equipment/materials
- ☐ Get an Andameds account
- ☐ Get an Amazon Business account
- ☐ Get a business bank account

Protect Yourself

- ☐ Purchase malpractice coverage
- ☐ Affirm pharmacy regulations and license requirements in your state
- ☐ Submit CLIA waiver
- ☐ Review HIPAA requirements and make sure emails and website are compliant.
- ☐ Write your patient contract.
- ☐ Finalize radiology, medication and lab agreements and sign BAA's.

- [ ] Finalize EMR, billing and other technology and sign/get BAA's.
- [ ] Decide on Medicare and submit opt-out application if needed
- [ ] Begin purchasing supplies

Final Touches
-1 month out-

- [ ] Finish/build out your website
- [ ] Generate a welcome to the practice letter
- [ ] Generate clinic policies-patient termination, billing, contracting, narcotic policies, nursing contracts, vacation policies and agreements.
- [ ] Think about access, texting, after hours, setting expectations for patients.
- [ ] Generate and send a letter to local small business owners
- [ ] Order your supplies and medications

- [ ] Begin scheduling
- [ ] Put in your vacation time (holds)

- [ ] Get lab supplies delivered including computer if needed, centrifuge, set up courier timing/agreements.
- [ ] Do a test run on blood, imaging, Rxs and patient sign up so you understand how things work.

Schedule ribbon cutting/opening party.

Open!

Step 1: What is your Vision?

If you know you want to do something different, then you have a vision. Let's work on defining it a little bit.

What does doctoring look like-- down to the color of the carpet and the chair in your waiting room-- what does it look like when you do it the way you've imagined? (You can write some notes here. Or start a Pinterest board!)

I'll come back to this a few more times in the next 19 steps. And you've kind of/sort of, already been jotting down 'vision notes'.

But write it down here, below: What's your vision?

More space: draw, scribble, tape in some pictures- what does a great day in a great place with a great team look like?

Step 2: Budget, Dave Ramsey style.

Dave Ramsey is a very conservative financial guru. You can learn a whole lot from him. But I'll save you time for now. Get your finances in order.

You need to figure out how much you spend, every month. When you know what you spend, you know what you need to earn.

Pull your bank account, credit cards etc... average out your spending over the last 12 months. On the next page is our spreadsheet in the event it will help. The first column, "current" is for you to jot down your rough numbers. After you have a rough spreadsheet, pull credit card statements or bank accounts and make it accurate. Figure out what you spend. You can keep things like your mortgage, childcare etc on credit cards but everything else... any and all elective spending-- go to cash. Figure out what you are spending and what you want to spend and start with a cash budget.

Get 5-10 envelopes. And label them:

a) my personal spending b) your partner's personal spending c) family fun (for all elective family fun- eating out, movies, etc) d) groceries, e) kids elective money/spending f) transportation/gas -- basically, make an envelope for anything you spend that you do not HAVE to spend. Set a budget for each envelope for a month and see if you can stick to it.

At the middle of the first month when you run out, revise.

Repeat x 3 months...

Home Budget
2017 Financial Projection

	Current	January	February	March
Net Income (after taxes, 401k, health insurance, etc.)				
Practice		$0	$0	$0
Side job 1		$4,000	$4,000	$4,000
Side job 2		$2,000	$2,000	$2,000
Spouse/significant other		$5,000	$5,000	$5,000
Bonus/other		$0	$0	$5,000
Total		$11,000	$11,000	$16,000
Expenses				
Mortgage		$1,800	$1,800	$1,800
Life Insurance		$1,000	$1,000	$1,000
Kids school		$1,100	$1,100	$1,100
Car payment(s)		$400	$400	$400
Student loan 1		$180	$180	$180
Student loan 2		$725	$725	$725
Groceries		$1,200	$1,200	$1,200
Eating Out		$700	$700	$700
Home phone/Internet		$100	$100	$100
Natural gas		$150	$150	$150
Water		$45	$50	$75
Electricity		$90	$90	$90
City Utilities		$25	$25	$25
Personal Cell Phones		$90	$90	$90
House Improvements Budget		$100	$100	$100
Family Necessities/Entertainment		400	$400	$400
Owner Contribution to practice		$0	$0	$2,000
Buffer		$1,000	$1,000	$1,000
Total		$9,105	$9,110	$11,135
Net Cash Flow		$1,895	$1,890	$4,865
Bank account after				
Net cash flow change		$11,895	$13,785	$18,650
Other deposits		$0	$0	$0
Other withdrawals (negative)		$0	$0	$0
Total	$10,000	$11,895	$13,785	$18,650

After 3 months we found that the budget that made sense on paper didn't work. Our 'sounds great' budget and our 'I can live with this' budget were different. We needed to increase our month to month cash amount which meant we wouldn't be able to start our practice on the timeline we wanted. (Or ever, actually). So we looked at what we could give up. Turns out it was our house.

We sold our house, our truck, turned in our two leased vehicles, cancelled gym memberships and subscription services (TV, lawn care) and bought a smaller house in the same school district a mile away and leased two base model vehicles. This freed up about $1400/month in previously fixed expenses and generated $20,000 for a start up nest egg.

You have to figure out what you HAVE and then you can work on making what you WANT.

Draft out your expenses for the next five years along with your income sources. This creates the groundwork for something called a 'proforma' that bankers and folks might want in a few months as you work on your business vision. It also helps you figure out if you can make this work.

Take your corrected Dave Ramsey style budgeting, now that you know it is pretty accurate and copy it out for the next 5 years. Add in known potential expenses- school, travel, vacations, new house, new car, buffer for unexpected things (healthcare!). Map out what you know you NEED.

Step 3: Create a safety net (aka get a side job).

After you've lived with a cash budget for three to four months you will have a much more transparent sense of what you can and cannot do within that time frame. Here's a small business pearl: 50% of all small businesses fail in the first year. And 50% of those that remain, will fail within the first 3 years. Why do they fail? (there are whole professions about this)-- in my opinion? A crappy business plan and/or too much overhead. (This is why buying a building starting out is dangerous).

So, create a safety net. Figure out how you will make money while you're not making money. Sequester resources.

Here's way to build/have a safety net

1. Work your tail off in the year prior to leaving and take advantage of financial bonus structures. You may keep more money in your pocket by starting to purchase items for your business and working with an accountant to write these expenses off.

2. If you are in a position to negotiate a different job out of your present work circumstance, (if you can disclose to your present employer that you will be changing circumstances), can you transition to urgent care/part time/locums/coverage within your current employment situation? What about being paid for call coverage? etc...

3. Get a side job. There are innumerable jobs for physicians that pay quite well and demand work that you can do at night, on weekends, and in between urgent care patients. I STRONGLY believe it is best to negotiate an HOURLY wage in these scenarios ($100-$250/hour or daily per diem of $1200-$2500+). The reason for the hourly wage is your mental health. When you are a 'fill in' doctor, you lose some leverage and gain some leverage. Your leverage is helping get clinics out of 'coverage binds'. Meaning, if you can offer last-minute flexibility, you have an opportunity. But the more the clinic needs PRN coverage, the more likely the clinic is REALLY dysfunctional. Which means you'll be double/triple booked, over-booked, booked after the day is over, etc… The EMR will be terrible and you will have no control. So, negotiate an hourly wage. A patient walk in at 5pm that keeps you there an hour --extra-cha-ching! EMR goes down and you have to 're-do' your notes (say no!! But if you can't, cha-ching.) Other than doing my own thing, nothing has been better for my mental health than being paid a competitive hourly wage. Bring. It. On. Because you know what? It's money in the bank for your vision!

Phil Eskew is a lawyer, an MBA and a physician. And he is a DPC rockstar. No one knows more about side-jobs in DPC than Phil. Actually, I'd bet no one knows more about DPC than Phil. Use his website: **www.dpcfrontier.com**.

Here are a few ideas of side jobs other DPC physicians have had while they built their practice. Now, mind you, which ones of these make the most sense for you does depend on what you decide to do with Medicare. We'll talk about that in a minute.

1. Working at/for a correctional facility (quite geographic dependent). Works with Medicare opt-out status and pays pretty well.
2. Doing life insurance exams: sporadic, doesn't pay much ~$90/hour, works with opt out status.
3. Moonlighting at an ER: there are ways to structure this if you are opted out because an exception is made for emergency care. You can do your clinic work in between patients (sometimes), keeps you on medical staff/connections at the hospital. ? Opportunity to market your practice. hourly rate is very high/competitive depending on situation/market
4. Working at an Urgent Care or on-site employee clinic: if you're efficient you can do your other work simultaneously. May work with opt-out situations depending on how billing is done/if there are medicare beneficiaries being seen, generally an hourly rate $100-$150/hour for an MD depending on market
5. Hospice medical directorship: Per medicare guidelines, billing is done under the hospice medical director who can designate to other MD/DO's that they are 'associates'. Payment is often salaried/contract rate hourly. Hospice medical directorships, as long as NO Medicare billing is done in your name is an opt-out eligible job. And it can be a win-win because many hospices just need an MD/DO three or five or ten

hours per week. Again, systems are not super open to thinking about this creatively, sometimes. This is a mostly administrative job with occasional face to face meetings. You're already on call, why not be on call and get paid? (hourly rate should be $130-$250 depending on your market).

6. VES (Veterans Affairs evaluations): helping with backlog of service-connected/disability evals. Scheduling per your availability. Need a physical location that is handicap accessible. Works with medicare opt out situation. Pay is about $40/30mins, variable. Lots of paperwork but pretty algorithmic

7. Locum tenens with an agency such as Goldfish partners. You can fly-in one week/month in some markets. Range seems to be $70-90/hour for UC/ER. True locums tenens work is billed in the name of the person the locum is covering for so it can be done in medicare-opt out situation. However, anything scheduled/habitual or lasting more than 6 months is technically not locums.

8. Filling in/covering for a physician out on medical/maternity leave. Ask around your medical community. There are likely independent MDs who need some type of coverage

9. Reviewing charts for an insurance company (ha!-- but it's an option... and if it pays, it's the most thematically Robin Hood form of getting a DPC practice going!)

10. Expert testimony (please work on behalf of physicians) can generate an hourly wage up to $300-$400! And often it's work you can do on your own schedule. They're docs in the DPC community who do this work who are happy to

share their experience. SEAK is another company that maintains a database of non-clinical opportunities for physicians.
11. Be creative! You have SO much to offer.

Step 4: Educate Yourself.

Resources include google, www.dpcfrontier.com,
www.dpcare.com, www.atlas.md, www.forbes.com,
www.aafp.com and a whole host of other resources.
Douglas Farrago, MD maintains a blog (authentic
medicine.com), is a practicing DPC physician and
published a comprehensive how to start your own DPC
clinic book in 2016. It's available on Amazon (The
Official Guide to Starting Your Own Direct Primary Care
Practice) and is a great place to start. Dr Paul Thomas's
DPC book, Direct Primary Care: The Cure for Our
Broken Healthcare System. Take some time, maybe
about 20 hours... and read everything you can get your
hands on about direct primary care and innovative
practice models. (Please, please, please make an effort to
inform yourself as you also lean on the DPC
community!)

There are great networking opportunities for DPC
annually including the AAFP DPC Summit held in
June/July of each year, the Hint Summit, usually in
April/May, and assorted events hosted by AAPP, AAPS
or FMEC. These are SUPERB places to network, and to
fill your brain with what is earnestly about $10,000 in
consulting input. Take the time to go to these
conferences, especially in the beginning.
Dr/Lawyer/MBA Phil Eskew maintains an up to date
"DPC" event list on his website, www.dpcfrontier.com.

Step 5: Haves & Needs: What Barriers Exist?

Review the terms of your existing contract for bonus payback terms, non-compete clauses, and assess for opportunities for re-negotiation while you're still 'in the game'. Even better-- never, never, never sign a contract with a non-compete or a restricted service area.

Step 6: Haves and Needs: What Do You Need and How Can You Get It?

While you're employed-what can you leverage?

- Can you work hard for 6 months, get a huge bonus and use that as start-up funds?
- Can you sell your house, cars, re-arrange your financial life and lean on your spouse as you build?
- Can you change the terms of your employment contract with your private practice in mind?
- Can you change your job entirely to a locums, weekend, night, ER, hospice, prison job -- a job that would provide transitional opportunities while you build your practice?
- Can you negotiate out of a non-compete with the hospital CEO or change the game and continue to do hospitalist work without charging a physician fee?
- Can you raise venture capital funding?
- Do you have someone you know who would be an investor in your practice by providing a low interest loan?

ALL of these have been done by DPC doctors currently running successful practices.

Dr. Vance Lassey owns Holton Direct Care in Holton, Kansas. He is a master at getting things done himself, for free or for trade. He was also able to negotiate a way to continue to do hospitalist work while opening a DPC practice. Dr. Vance provided the following recommendations and insights into how to build a medical clinic on a dime and a prayer.

Finding Steals and Making Deals
How to Save Money Starting Your Direct Primary Care Clinic
By Vance Lassey, MD

Part One: Introduction and Basic Principles

If you have a wealthy benefactor, a trust fund, or otherwise have money to spend at your leisure, enjoy the ease of your DPC startup, and please feel free to skip this article, and know that the rest of us expect you to buy our dinner and drinks at the next DPC conference.

We doctors generally have decades of scientific education, but little to no education about business or money. I had ZERO business knowledge, but I *knew* I had to DPC so I jumped in, and I learned as I went. The good news, is that most of this really turns out to be common sense.

The first thing to know is that you're going to have to keep your overhead down if you ever want to make money again. One good way to keep your overhead down is to avoid interest payments. That means starting up without a loan if you can. This is possible, but rarely so without major sacrifice. But, **starting a clinic doesn't have to cost a fortune**, so look at your situation and see if you can make a no-loan startup a reality. Zoom out as far as you can and make some over-arching assessments of your financial situation, and your goals. Then, make yourself a few guiding principles and boundaries, follow them as much as possible, and the solution should present itself.

I'll demonstrate this by using my own goal, assessments, and solution (yours will be different, of course).

> **Goal:** Be self-employed ASAP. Pure DPC. Doing medicine right and having time for my patients, family, and self is more important than my income, and when this works, the money will follow.

> **Assessment 1:** I owed some money on my house and my 115 acre farm. But not *that* much. Otherwise, I

was almost out of debt, and want to get all the way out.

Assessment 2: I was so dedicated to my DPC goals, that I was willing to make painful sacrifices to achieve them.

Principle 1: No loans. I hate paying interest, and don't want to go into debt.

Principle 2: No/Minimal moonlighting. After 9 very long years on the inside, I was due for some much-needed time for my family and my physical and mental health.

Solution: Liquidate. I sold about ⅔ of the farm I'd killed myself working on the inside for 9 years to buy. That was my sacrifice, and it hurt. But, the sting of letting go of it was short lived, and the deep breath of fresh air on the outside of the system was more than worth it. And, with the tidy profit on the sale, I paid off all my outstanding debt, and put some money in the bank, enough for us to live on for a year or two if we budget tightly, and pay for my clinic's startup costs *as long as they would be kept LOW.* And now I have zero debt, which is a good place to be if you're starting *any* business.

So that's how I started a clinic without a loan. But I had equity I could liquidate. The alternative (taking out a loan) is often chosen, sometimes by necessity. This requires income to pay interest on your loan. Assuming you don't ramp up your clinic overnight, you're going to find yourself moonlighting all the time to pay for all this, and if your business fails, you're hosed. I'm not saying there's anything wrong with this approach, but one of the things that is attractive about DPC is that you no longer work 7 days a week away from your family. If you're running your new business M-F and moonlighting at nights and on weekends to pay for it while it ramps up, you're not much better off than you were before. That being said, such pain is temporary, and doing this requires a sacrifice in every case. If that is the sacrifice you must make, then make it. The rough schedule will motivate you to strive all the more to be successful and gain independence in DPC. There are numerous ways to make money on the side while your DPC clinic ramps up, but that is not the focus of this article.

If you've got no choice to go into debt to start your clinic, you're still much better off starting the clinic on a very strict budget. It is not difficult to spend hundreds of thousands starting a clinic, and then remain a slave to the bank for years and years to pay it off. Get a line of credit, and use only what you have to, because the smaller the loan, the smaller the payments and the more quickly you'll be able to pay it off and become a profitable business. Including paying my nurse a full salary for 3 months before we opened, I was able to start my clinic for under $30,000, and I've heard of others doing it for even less. I made all that back in a few months and was in the black in no time, with no loan and no moonlighting.

Don't forget to live on a tight budget. Income is thin for a while while you ramp up. If you don't want to burn yourself down working multiple side-jobs, it helps to get yourself out of debt ASAP. Sell fancy cars, buy a used car. If you are paying off a mortgage on a big house, sell it and downsize to something you can pay cash for with the money. Clip coupons and don't shop at Whole Foods. Then you can live in low-stress peace with your weekends off, with 100% of your time available to give your own business as you build it and ramp up. When you've got a successful DPC clinic and have become financially comfortable in a few years, knock yourself out. Delay gratification.

Part 2: Medical Inflation: The main reason I had to write this article.

In medicine, the cost of everything has become hyper-inflated. Stupid hyper-inflated. Maybe this will get better as a result of our efforts in free-market medicine, but until it does, we have to deal with it. The problem we have in DPC is that the over-pricing in medicine has trickled down to the suppliers and wholesalers, too. If they sell an office chair to a business office, the cost is, say $100. But if it's medical supply, they take the same chair, label it a *nurse's chair*, and list it for $350. But can you blame them? If a clinic is charging patients $75 for a $3 CBC, the "medical furniture" place can justifiably gouge the clinic for an office chair. But if you're in DPC and you sell that CBC for $3, you need to avoid being gouged, so you won't be forced to pass these costs on to your patients.

Part 3: Cost-Savings Pearls

1) Get as much free stuff as you can.
Of course I'm going to be talking about getting cheap or used stuff, but why stop there? Why not go for *free* stuff? As an example: I found a non-profit hospital, and approached the guy in charge of their materials management department. I asked him about surplus stuff--anything they might have--and asked if he would be interested in selling it at low prices to a clinic that was going to be caring for lots of uninsured people, etc. He said that as a non-profit, he couldn't sell it, but that much of their surplus inventory was going to be thrown away and I could have about anything I wanted, *for free*. I got a like-new electric exam table, a power procedure table, an autoclave, numerous cabinets, office chairs, waiting room chairs, paper towel dispensers, glove box holders, a scale, a lab-drawing chair, wall-mounted otoscope/opthalmascope, countertops, curtain track, halogen exam light, physician's exam stools and more. Buying that stuff new would have cost me thousands. Who cares if it's used? Clean it up, slap a coat of paint on it where necessary, and count your savings.

2) Get Free Advice and whenever possible, *Figure It Out*.
Don't forget more than just *stuff* can be free. Advice can also be free. There are plenty of opportunists who will try to get you to buy services or advice from them, or attend for-profit seminars or boot camps, and they'll do everything they can to convince you that without their magic knowledge and service you're going to fail. They'll tell you they can help you build your practice, teach you how to start a business, do your marketing, design your website for you, etc. They'll even promise you a certain rate of growth, as if they have any control on that! This is all bogus. *These services or advice are available elsewhere*

for free. Just because you've never designed a website, marketed a business, set up an internet domain, done the financial books on a business, or whatever it may be doesn't mean you need to pay some schmuck thousands to do it for you. *Figure out how to do it and do it yourself.* With advice, there are scores of DPC docs out there in numerous online forums who have gone before you who would gladly give you free advice. Don't fall for all these scams. They're everywhere--people who want to take your energetic leap into business and suck it dry. Parasites, the lot of them.

3) Get used stuff, cheap.
This is huge. Don't buy anything new unless you have no other option. Don't buy surgical instruments from surgical supply stores, because they gouge you hard. Instead, hit up eBay and Craigslist. I use hemoclips in my vasectomies, and the clip appliers from supply places were like $150-200 as I recall. I got a like new Ethicon clip applier on eBay for $10. I got a pristine ConMed Hyfrecator last week for $350 on eBay, which is something like $800 new. Another option is to find clinics/hospitals that are closing, and contact them about buying used stuff. It's all surplus to them, and hard to sell much of it, so you can cash in. Call your state medical society and ask about clinics that are closing. Keep your eyes out for auctions and go to as many as you can. I'm not just talking medical auctions. You can find furniture, cabinets, wire storage shelving, wall art, and much much more. I went to an auction at a hotel that had gone out of business. There, I nabbed a big stainless steel wire storage rack, probably worth at least $250 new, for $1. At the same auction I got a big UPS worth hundreds (to keep computers on in case of power failure) for $0.50, a new mini-fridge for $20 that I keep insulin in, and a break room microwave for $3. Never know what you'll find, but you can get amazing deals.

4) Get your hands dirty.
Manual labor is the most expensive thing you'll buy if you're building or renovating anything. In my small clinic, the materials for the somewhat extensive renovation were approximately $4,000. My Dad and I spent over 720 hours (combined) over about 6 weeks doing all the work ourselves.

That labor would have cost me well over $15,000, and it might have been shoddy work. *Lack of experience is a lousy excuse for not doing this.* If you can learn to perform surgery on a human being, you can learn to lay bathroom tile, install a sink, or refinish window trim. Watch a YouTube video and learn how to do the work. It's not hard, and if you're willing to invest sweat equity, the dividends will be massive.

5) Renting? Negotiate to get paid for your labor!
On top of your labor savings, if you're renting, you can negotiate the value of your labor against the value of your upcoming rent, since you're fixing up the owner's building. In the case of my clinic, the building owner felt that he can rent it for way more after I leave in a couple years (when I build my dedicated clinic) because it's way nicer than it used to be, and that's worth something to him. We crunched numbers and figured that the value of my labor offsets my rent and utilities for 2 years. So I spent 6 weeks busting my butt fixing up the place, and now I don't pay rent or utilities for 2 years. If you're absolutely unwilling to do manual labor, then barter for it. Find a builder who is getting robbed on his health care, and trade him a year or two of care in exchange for renovating your clinic. And since you're the one paying him (in medical services) for the work, you can then barter with the landlord for a couple years of rent in exchange for increasing the value and rentability of his or her facility. With that smart deal, you get free rent AND free renovation labor. More on bartering coming up.

6) Make your labor a valuable (but free) advertisement.
Another neat thing about doing the work myself, is it gave me a huge selling point on facebook, where I did all my own (free) advertising. Occasionally I'd post pictures of myself covered in paint or sheetrock mud, patching up walls or a time lapse video I made of me laying flooring. The tagline on every post went something like "If I don't have to pay somebody to install this floor, neither do my patients. Welcome to Direct Primary Care." The patients get that. You're saving *them* money. That's effective marketing, it's true, and it's free. Plus, patients like having a doctor who's a human being, and your humility, work

ethic, and idealism (you're doing this to save *them* money) is a valuable selling point.

7) Bartering. This one is a little bit tricky, but has it's place. When you trade for goods and services, both parties need to feel like they're getting a good deal. This never works otherwise. Value is in the eye of the beholder. If you can't both agree that your deal makes sense to you both, switch back to using money. Josh Umbehr once told me "You can both always agree on the value of a dollar." I had a farmer who wanted to trade me about $400 worth of beef for about $1000 worth of membership fees. But my freezer was already full. Obviously, I didn't like the deal. (Luckily he found out that I could save him over $120 monthly on his meds which more than offset his $100 membership and we didn't have to keep having the beef negotiation!) But perhaps you could give a housekeeper free membership in exchange for his or her services. When you take a social history and your new patient tells you he's a computer/IT specialist at your local bank, ask him if he'd ever be interested in trading a month's membership fee when you need your computer fixed. Probably will only take him 15 minutes, and saves you a bundle--you both win. Bartering is generally a no-money traded affair, but you're trading goods or services with a monetary value. For this reason, you need to agree on monetary value of the traded services and keep records for tax purposes- this is something to discuss with your accountant.

	HAS	DOESN'T HAVE / NEEDS
DOCTOR	Excellent Medical Care to give	Rent-free Clinic Space
LANDLORD	Building to Rent in need of remodeling	Time/$ to Remodel
BUILDER	Time and Skills to Remodel	Quality Health Care

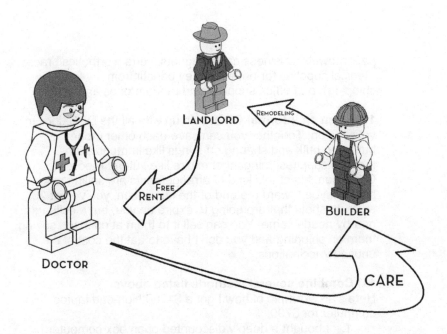

LANDLORD

REMODELING

FREE
RENT

BUILDER

DOCTOR

CARE

8) Ask others.
You're not the first person to start a DPC clinic on a dime. When you can't figure out the cheap way to do something, ask somebody who's been there before you. There are online groups, discussion forums, even books. Many DPC docs have come up with novel ways to save money.

9) Join a GPO.
Group Purchasing Organizations are basically like a discount membership. You pay a fee or buy a product (such as an EMR, for instance) and with it comes discounts at places that sell stuff you might need. (Medication wholesalers, medical equipment suppliers, wholesale labs/pathology services, etc.) If you can't get the thing you need anywhere else, and you're stuck getting it from a supplier, you might as well be part of a GPO so you get a group discount. Along these lines, get Amazon prime. $100 a year gets you free shipping on most stuff from Amazon.com, and often you can get things there at lower prices even than your wholesale suppliers, or suppliers in your GPO. Things I get there include

paper towels, business card magnets, certain orthotics/braces, medical supplies for patients (they benefit from my free shipping), and office supplies and random odds and ends.

10) Form an informal GPO. Join up with all the DPC docs in your region. Together you can save each other money by buying in bulk and sharing on things like immunizations, medical supplies, things that expire like suture, meds, etc. Other benefits of this kind of arrangements are selling extra stuff. Maybe toward the end of the flu season, you've got 20 extra flu shots that are going to expire on you, but a colleague nearby needs some. You can sell it to them at cost and saving them on shipping and you don't have to eat the cost of the unused vaccinations.

11) Combine several methods listed above.
Here's an example of how I got a $1300 high-end laptop computer for $700:
1. I bought a deeply discounted open box computer online. This computer did not come with the manufacturer or retailer's warranty-- a risky purchase if you aren't a computer guru. As suspected, the like-new computer had been registered and passworded, etc. by the original owner, so it didn't work.
2. My patient who works at the bank and is a computer/IT guru traded me 2 months worth of care (a $60 value) and he spent about an hour fully wiping this computer and re-installing all the software. Now it's as good as new, super-fast, very powerful, and basically I got it for half price.

Starting a DPC clinic doesn't have to be incredibly expensive, but it is if you're not willing to be creative, look for deals, find mentors, and negotiate wherever possible. Regardless of how you go about it, **do it.** DPC is incredibly rewarding!

Step 7: Haves & Needs: Get a Mentor.

EVERY entrepreneur needs a mentor. Remember all of
that self-education you did? Pick out three to five people
whose message, model or mission really resonates with
you and contact them. See if you can visit their clinic.
Get out of your doctor box and get as much exposure as
you can to people who are doing what you do.

On that note, you are probably feeling excited. (I'm
excited!) Look at all of this concrete guidance about how
to build your own clinic.

But, what is it really like?

Most DPC docs will tell you that they are very, very
happy. They have autonomy. They get to spend time with
patients. The feel like DOCTORS. There's no one
breathing down their back to get notes, or coding, or
compliance matters or EMR training done. Most DPC
docs will also tell you that they're tired. Really tired.
DPC is not easier. It's not less work. It's different work.
If your interest in DPC is to make more than $200K and
work less, good luck. That is *some* DPC doctors
experience. But most of us are putting in 60-70-80 hours.
They are (mostly) joyful hours.

Dr. Nicholas Tomsen owns Antioch Med, a DPC practice
in Wichita, Kansas. He opened July 11, 2016. Here's how
he describes a somewhat typical day.

5/30/17

Antioch Med - a day in the life. Currently 470 patients, open 10.5 months.

- 12 total visits (day after a holiday weekend though): 2 procedures (toenail, lesion removal), 4 follow up visits, 5 acute visits, 1 home visit and 1 new patient.
- 74 total technology "touches" (either sent or received message: text, email, voicemail)
- Prescriptions filled: 17 individual prescriptions, 471 total pills, 1 IM injection
- Order: One x-ray ordered
- Labs drawn: 2 sets

7:30 AM arrived to the office and review the day's schedule and emailed 3 patients their lab results for chronic disease management - CKD, HTN, HLD, DMII, anemia workup. Huddled with my nurse about tasks that needed done for the day, follow up from the weekend that needed done, and medications that needed to be ordered.
8 Follow up visit for weight reduction/phentermine management
8:30 Follow up - teenager with tibial stress fracture and female athlete triad
9 Sister of the 16 yr old wanted a lesion on her leg removed, so we removed it :)
9:30 New patient - uninsured and in 20s with history of anemia and GI symptoms. Beginning workup for IBD
10:30 Acute visit 30 yr old with a rash on her face (hairdresser with contact dermatitis). Also informed me that she and her husband are planning on getting pregnant soon and talked about fertility monitoring and pre-conception counseling. Husband at the end of the visit states that he has been having more depressive symptoms (history of schizophrenia that I co-manage with psychiatry). Called psychiatrist and scheduled him to follow up in 2 days and scheduled initial visit for counseling. He is texting me updates weekly regarding his follow up.
11:30-1 PM Ate lunch with friends nearby and caught upon text messages and emails.
1 Toenail removal in the office
1:30 Follow up pneumonia, hypothyroidism with recent myxedema, discussed smoking cessation
2 Follow up on anxiety in patient with IBS and probable panic attacks.
2:30 Acute visit for sinusitis in patient with prior sinus cancer and chronic radiation related facial damage
2:45 Acute visit for pyelonephritis (told me that I saved her life at the end of the visit and started crying - not because of treating her it i but because she is now 5 months off of narcotics with our help after previously being on nearly 100 mg oxycodone in a day for the last 5 years!)
4 Acute visit for suspected boxer fracture from Memorial Day Shenanigans :)
4:30 Acute visit for pharyngitis, strep negative
5 Acute home visit: abdominal pain, N/V/D, hypovolemia. IVF given at the house (IV that I started - boom). Lab drawn and antiemetics given.
6:30 Home with my family:)

In general, this is a busier day than usual for me, but not unexpected following the holiday weekend and about par for me for a very busy day. I work in general 8 half days of the week seeing patients, 1 half day doing admin, and one half day off with my kids. I have one full time nurse that both she and I answer the phone, draw labs, dispense meds, reply to texts, clean rooms, etc. We were running hard this day, but no one was rushed out of the office and everyone felt cared for. I got ¾ of my notes done in that time and the rest done the following morning that was slower. -Nick

Step 8: Haves & Needs: Build a Team.

You can do this. You need a mentor, a supportive partner and small business contacts.

Many, in fact, a vast majority of DPC doctors have incredibly supportive partners. It's not uncommon among the smaller/solo clinics for a husband-wife (or wife-wife or husband-husband) team to work together. If your partner is not on board with your vision, this is going to be very difficult. Take your partner to a DPC conference...let them see what it is you are talking about. If they live with you and all of your exhausted, disillusioned burn out, I have no doubt they'll come along as you build your DPC vision. And...if they don't/won't/can't... You've got some big decisions to make.

As you build your team, consider joining a small business group- whether BNI ("Business Networking international") or your local Chamber of Commerce or both. Your best mentor may be a twenty-eight year old real estate magnate. Consider reaching out to an accountant, a commercial real estate agent, a lawyer, a graphic designer and a web-designer as you start to lay the groundwork for your business. (As you do, remember, these folks have a lot of connections.) Ask for a thirty minute interview at no charge to explain your needs and to see if they are the right fit. Learn how to sell your idea early on because these very well may be some of your best future referral sources!

Step 9: Building a Brand.

A brand is a promise.

Pretty soon you're going to need to write a business plan. And even if you don't NEED it, the process of creating it will help you grow as a business person and to refine your vision. Business plans are difficult. They take a long time.

Your business plan is where you are going to clarify your message and make this whole vision make sense on paper. If you need money, your business plan is how you're going to get it. Remember the first baby you delivered (the horror!)? Much harder. You can do this. Here's how:

a.   You are now a doctor *and* a small business entrepreneur. The next few years are going to be filled with learning about small business and business ownership. I'll tell you right now- many physicians are weird. We train in a box. We don't learn how to negotiate, sell, and communicate the way many of our non-doctor peers do. You have a lot to learn. Be humble. There are chiropractors and naturopaths and counsellors out there making millions yearly on healthcare. We might disagree with their healthcare discipline (or not), but they deserve credit for their business acumen.

b.   Remember the vision question? Here's why it matters. Businesses need a mission statement. Mission statements force you to figure out, simply, what your promise is. A branding expert taught me: "a brand matters. A brand is a promise."

What is your promise?

Ours was "the most straight-forward medical care you'll ever receive."

Yup, too long. Ok, how about- "no bullshit." (we found out that "no bullshit" is trademarked... and probably not family-medicine-PC).

Write it again, simplified.

And simplify it more.

*Ours: "direct, compassionate, high quality affordable healthcare" (damn. still too long). . . **and then we got to:** "healthcare. simplified'.*

There it is.

You've got your promise. Now you can plan.

What's in a name?

Shakespeare asked, "What's in a name?" While the name you choose is quite important, it is not nearly as important as the service you provide. Your service builds your brand and your brand reflects your service.

How do you decide what to call yourself?

Dr. Thomas White, one of my absolute favorite people on the planet, and an outstanding physician and DPC doc has said that, "maybe the best name is YOUR name." Don't fret too much as you try to figure out what to call yourself. In the beginning (and maybe forever), it just may be that YOUR name is the best name. If you want to come up with something different, there's lots of ways to do it.

We chose to NOT name our practice after me (Dr. Julie) because our vision was to have a few clinics with multiple physicians eventually. We wanted to figure out the model well enough to start to provide a place for inspired physicians to be employed and excited. We wanted something that signified change, the beginning of something different. Where we live, every summer, there are many, many forrest fires. Sparks start fires. That's how we ultimately came up with sparkMD. But it took some brainstorming.

Work with a partner, friend/spouse, etc to come up with a list of, say, ten names that would represent your practice. See if the URL's are available, use google to come up with all kinds of synonyms for what you want to call yourself. When you settle on three or four, have an informal dinner party with eight to ten friends. Let them drink a lot. Ask them to say the first thing that comes to mind when you tell them your business names. Let them bruise up your ideas and point out how your favorite one actually sounds like a bodily function. In the long term, that kind of social vetting will help you settle on a name, and a logo, that will reflect your vision to others.

And now, the logo!

It is worth spending some money (like $2000 or less) to have someone professional help you with your logo. I used Entermotion design in Wichita and it was a fabulous experience. Other resources include www.etsy.com, www.99designs.com... There are a number of open source design sites where you can get an affordable, meaningful logo that is done professionally. It will serve you well for a long time.

Whatever way you go, when you pay for a logo/branding package consider how many 'logo' edits your package includes (two-three is probably a good idea). Think about the colors you choose and don't make it overly complicated. It needs to be on web sites, Facebook pages, pens, T-shirts, business cards. It needs to reproduce well in black and white and be flexible enough to fit in square spaces, circle spaces and stretched rectangular spaces. Your logo doesn't have to have four stereotypical healthcare elements (heart, stethoscope, cross, shield). Again, what is your vision? What looks like that vision?

Here's communication and inspiration from our design process:

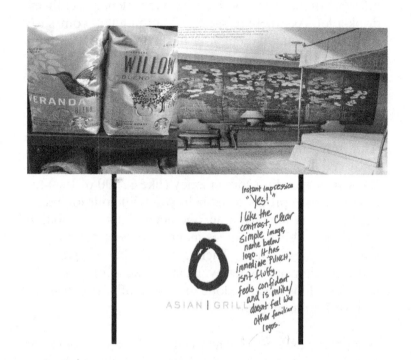

Instant impression
"Yes!"
I like the
contrast, clear
simple image
name below
logo. It has
immediate "PUNCH",
isn't fluffy,
feels confident
and is unlike/
doesn't feel like
other familiar
logos.

ASIAN | GRILL

And here were the three final logos:

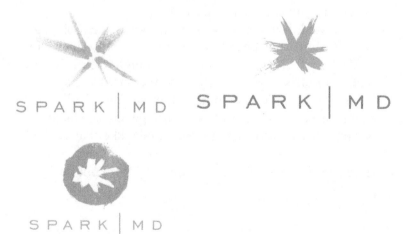

We picked the last one. The grey smudge is actually my thumbprint and the 'spark' is a spark and an asterisk*.

*because we always seem to keep the most important stuff hidden from plain sight.

A thought on branding:

As you demonstrate commitment to your mission, your brand builds and reinforces itself. Logos need to be recognizable to reinforce your brand but *your logo is not your brand*. Most of the world's major successful brands have very well-defined logos that can be cut down to one color and work well in black-and-white. Health programs are almost always muted colors or pastels. Food is red, orange and yellow. This doesn't mean you have to do muted colors and pastels but be mindful you don't recreate the big health insurance logos in feel and color.

I wouldn't want my direct primary care clinic which I'm trying to differentiate from the old guard to resonate a brand that people already know that is basically what we're saying doesn't work.

Making a logo is fun. It's creative. It feels like- yes!- I'm doing something for my business. People get GRADUATE degrees, even PhDs in design and spend just as much time building an expertise around branding as we spend training to be doctors. Branding is a *thing*. It matters. Hire an expert.

I'm sure this sounds a little complicated, or overwhelming, or maybe my priorities in terms of the visual arts are skewed. But, this is going to work. And what that means is you are going to be saying, using and handing out materials with this icon on it for the rest of your professional life. Put some effort into it. Get it right (or as right as you can), and use it to make a statement (which is what a logo should do, right?)

Step 10: Pick a Location.

A number of DPC docs say figuring out *where* they are going practice is one of the toughest parts of starting their practice. Specifically, finding the space, negotiating the pricing, planning around the build out (which is NEVER completed on time) and being ready to open is a source for stress. A few DPC docs said this stage needs at least 5 months time from finding space to being ready to open.

Considerations include needed square footage, type of access (stairs, elevator, ample parking?), other tenants, duration of your lease, whether or not the land-lord is willing to pay for the build-outs so your space is usable by you and if there is accessible plumbing. Other considerations are whether or not you can get 3-6 months 'free', and who takes care of the landscaping, cleaning, maintenance? Can you grow in this space (do you need to?) Is the space permitted for what you want to do? Would you rather own?

In general, most entrepreneurs will tell you to never, ever, ever buy a property at the start of your business. Keep your overhead LOW. A few DPC docs (I am one of them), however, have made small practice models work along with property ownership. Just figure out what your vision is, what you have, what you need, how much risk you can tolerate and how long you can go without a full income.

What community, clinic, space, environment- what location would help your business thrive?

There is NO data to support this but in 2014, when we were just about to open spark, someone at a DPC conference noted that many of the successful DPC practices at the time were within a 1-2 mile range of a Whole Foods grocery store. (I do not remember who provided this information but it stuck with me.) Lucky for us, we had bought a building within 6 blocks of the only Whole Foods in Idaho! In all seriousness, though, where I grew up- Idaho- there is a grocery conglomerate called "Albertsons". Throughout my childhood Albertsons' stores were opening all over the valley as our population grew. I recently learned that the CEO's of Albertsons and St. Alphonsus (one of the big hospital systems) were good friends. Albertsons would do incredible amounts of demographic research and then decide where to buy land, hold it, negotiate 'non-competes' of sorts to keep other grocers away and then eventually open a grocery store. St. Alphonsus purchased land where ever Albertson's did. . .

Study the DPC clinics that are successful. If you are opening in a place you know, think about who your audience is, where do they live, what do they need? Patients will drive quite a long ways for a good doctor. So pick a place that helps your business grow or a place that is within range of where you want your forever clinic to be.

Step 11: How Many & How Much?

Time for spreadsheets and figuring out your pricing

Now that you have your personal budget and you have your business plan (or most of it...) you've probably noticed that there's some number crunching we haven't discussed yet.

It's time to figure out the money and growth and patient census question that everyone wants to know about.

How many patients should I take care of?

How much should I charge?

There's a lot of ways to do this.

1. Dr. Forrest, a direct primary care innovator and physician out of Apex, North Carolina has recommended taking the number of patients you want to see per day and multiplying by 100 to get your panel size. He's also advised to take what you want to charge for your monthly fee, multiply it by the number of patients you want to have (minus 200 patients which in his model is the rough number needed to cover overhead) and that's your target take-home income.
2. MDVIP is a large corporate version of DPC (sort of) and they seem to think VERY strongly that this model taps out at 500.
3. MedLion previously would not permit you to have more than 1000 patients with their agreement.

4. AtlasMD and a number of other solo practices are built around a 600-800 patients/provider model.
5. And the good work of Dr. Phil Eskew demonstrated that the mean charge for DPC clinics in 2015 was $77/month.
6. As of the publication of this book there are no known updated studies regarding average monthly charges among the approximately 1300 DPC's nationally.

There are all kinds of ways to get to the right numbers for your vision. Here's how we got to our patient volume and pricing.

Our business promise was healthcare simplified. Our goal was to charge the least amount possible while still making a market-fair family medicine income AND accumulating an asset (remember I said we bought a building? That's the asset. I decided I wanted more than a watch after forty years of service.)

Our building cost: $450,000.

Our loans came out to ultimately be $4400/month for the building and build-out expenses. We did a big gut remodel. Two tenants' rent brought our cost to $3500/month. My nurse (with benefits etc) cost the practice $5000/month. My EMR $300/month. Malpractice insurance $~500/month. EMR/website fees $50/month. Our practice finance loan added $1200/month in loan pay backs. If I wanted to make my base plus have enough income for benefits, I needed (eventually) $15,000/month.

So, $3,500+ $5,000+ $300+ $500+ $50+ $1,200+
$1,5000 = $26,000 monthly.

Health insurance, electricity, cleaning, office supplies, lab
supplies etc... And I rounded this to $30,000.

Work and re-work your spreadsheet until you think
you're close. Then take that number and multiply it by
1.33 so you have a good margin of error. I did not do this
starting out.

With $30,000/month in overhead (when you figure in my
income) modelled out across various patient volumes:
$30,000/400= $75
$30,000/500= $60
$30,000/600= $50
$30,000/700= $43

We looked at this and thought about what our local
market would bear. This might have been a leap and is a
tough call if you don't know the area where you want to
open.

DPC Expenses, Sample

	Sample Month 1
Revenue	
Patient payments	$22,500
Pharmacy	$600
Owner contribution	$2,486
Total	$25,586
Expenses	
Salary and benefits (staff)	$4,068
Salary (Physician)	$0
Taxes (Payroll and IRS) - budget 30% of total salary pai	$1,120
Practice Loan (down payment)	$599
Practice Loan (working capital)	$799
Pharmacy Inventory (any rotating costs)	$0
EMR fees	$300
Misc Expenses	$2,500
Operations Expenses	$6,375
Lease	$2,000
Phones/Internet	$200
Gas/Heat	$100
Water	$125
Power Bills	$200
Accountant	$125
Electronic Faxing Company	$40
Malpractice Insurance	$1,000
Utilities	$15
Water District (other utilities)	$35
Landscaping/ground maintenance	$100
Lawyer Fees	$300
Advertising	$80
Liquid Nitrogen	$55
Unanticipated Expenses	$2,000
Total	$22,136
Net Cash Flow	$3,449
Bank account after	
Net cash flow change	$3,449
Other deposits	$0
Other withdrawals (negative)	$0
Total	$3,449

Then we took these numbers and thought about access-how much did we want to work? We found data that the average person sees a doctor 2.7 times/year (it's A LOT more in DPC, in our opinion!). We modeled out 5 visits/year and various scenarios - working 44, 45, 46, 47 weeks/year, 3.5 days, 4 days 4.5 days/week, having 8, 10, 14 visits/day. From our vision we knew we wanted quality time, quality relationships. We didn't want any visit to have to be less than 30 minutes. And we wanted 60 minutes for new patients.

Give yourself wiggle room for patients who don't pay (about 2% of our practice), patients who don't pay on time (about 5%), pipes that leak (yes, that happened), payroll taxes (damn, didn't know about those) and inflation.

We thought our model worked, tightly, at $50/month but we chose $60 because a business woman told it's much better to start a little high and NOT change prices for the start-up years than it is to undershoot and have an upward shifting price point in the middle of winning trust and business. After three years we announced we are raising our prices to $65/month for adults. And guess what? The vast majority of our patients asked why we weren't increasing the price more. In hindsight, we should have started at $75/month in our market for grown-ups. It would have made things A LOT less stressful.

At the end of the day, this is *not* a race to the bottom. The goal of DPC is to liberate yourself, liberate your patients and create a business model that is sustainable, and has both integrity and transparency in pricing. You can save patients a lot of money, hassle and time and not be stressed from paycheck to paycheck.

Patient volume tool (3 visits per patient per year)

J. Gunther 2017

		Gross	Net (after CC)
Weeks worked/year	46	Net monthly price/adult	$77.00 $74.69
Number of patient visits/year	3	Net monthly price/kids	$15.00 $14.55
Net margin (40% overhead)	60%		
Percentage adults	75%		
Percentage collected	98%		

Days worked/ week	Hours worked/ day	Average Visit Time	Visits per day	Total Available Visits	Patient Volume	Annual Revenue	Net Income
3	6	15	24	3312	1104	$774,503	$464,702
3	6	30	12	1656	552	$387,252	$232,351
3	6	45	8	1104	368	$258,168	$154,901
3	7	15	28	3864	1288	$903,587	$542,152
3	7	30	14	1932	644	$451,794	$271,076
3	7	45	9	1288	429	$301,196	$180,717
3	8	15	32	4416	1472	$1,032,671	$619,603
3	8	30	16	2208	736	$516,336	$309,801
3	8	45	11	1472	491	$344,224	$206,534
4	6	15	24	4416	1472	$1,032,671	$619,603
4	6	30	12	2208	736	$516,336	$309,801
4	6	45	8	1472	491	$344,224	$206,534
4	7	15	28	5152	1717	$1,204,783	$722,870
4	7	30	14	2576	859	$602,391	$361,435
4	7	45	9	1717	572	$401,594	$240,957
4	8	15	32	5888	1963	$1,376,895	$826,137
4	8	30	16	2944	981	$688,447	$413,068
4	8	45	11	1963	654	$458,965	$275,379
5	6	15	24	5520	1840	$1,290,839	$774,503
5	6	30	12	2760	920	$645,419	$387,252
5	6	45	8	1840	613	$430,280	$258,168
5	7	15	28	6440	2147	$1,505,979	$903,587
5	7	30	14	3220	1073	$752,989	$451,794
5	7	45	9	2147	716	$501,993	$301,196
5	8	15	32	7360	2453	$1,721,118	$1,032,671
5	8	30	16	3680	1227	$860,559	$516,336
5	8	45	11	2453	818	$573,706	$344,224

Patient volume tool (4 visits per patient per year)

						Gross	Net (after CC)
Weeks worked/year			46	Net monthly price/adult		$77.00	$74.69
Number of patient visits/year			4	Net monthly price/kids		$15.00	$14.55
Net margin (40% overhead)			60%				
Percentage adults			75%				
Percentage collected			98%				

Days worked/week	Hours worked/day	Average Visit Time	Visits per day	Total Available Visits	Patient Volume	Annual Revenue	Net Income
3	6	15	24	3312	828	$580,877	$348,526
3	6	30	12	1656	414	$290,439	$174,263
3	6	45	8	1104	276	$193,626	$116,175
3	7	15	28	3864	966	$677,690	$406,614
3	7	30	14	1932	483	$338,845	$203,307
3	7	45	9	1288	322	$225,897	$135,538
3	8	15	32	4416	1104	$774,503	$464,702
3	8	30	16	2208	552	$387,252	$232,351
3	8	45	11	1472	368	$258,168	$154,901
4	6	15	24	4416	1104	$774,503	$464,702
4	6	30	12	2208	552	$387,252	$232,351
4	6	45	8	1472	368	$258,168	$154,901
4	7	15	28	5152	1288	$903,587	$542,152
4	7	30	14	2576	644	$451,794	$271,076
4	7	45	9	1717	429	$301,196	$180,717
4	8	15	32	5888	1472	$1,032,671	$619,603
4	8	30	16	2944	736	$516,336	$309,801
4	8	45	11	1963	491	$344,224	$206,534
5	6	15	24	5520	1380	$968,129	$580,877
5	6	30	12	2760	690	$484,065	$290,439
5	6	45	8	1840	460	$322,710	$193,626
5	7	15	28	6440	1610	$1,129,484	$677,690
5	7	30	14	3220	805	$564,742	$338,845
5	7	45	9	2147	537	$376,495	$225,897
5	8	15	32	7360	1840	$1,290,839	$774,503
5	8	30	16	3680	920	$645,419	$387,252
5	8	45	11	2453	613	$430,280	$258,168

Patient volume tool (5 visits per patient per year)

J. Gunther 2017

						Gross	Net (after CC)
Weeks worked/year			46	Net monthly price/adult		$77.00	$74.69
Number of patient visits/year			5	Net monthly price/kids		$15.00	$14.55
Net margin (40% overhead)			60%				
Percentage adults			75%				
Percentage collected			98%				

Days worked/ week	Hours worked/ day	Average Visit Time	Visits per day	Total Available Visits	Patient Volume	Annual Revenue	Net Income
3	6	15	24	3312	662	$464,702	$278,821
3	6	30	12	1656	331	$232,351	$139,411
3	6	45	8	1104	221	$154,901	$92,940
3	7	15	28	3864	773	$542,152	$325,291
3	7	30	14	1932	386	$271,076	$162,646
3	7	45	9	1288	258	$180,717	$108,430
3	8	15	32	4416	883	$619,603	$371,762
3	8	30	16	2208	442	$309,801	$185,881
3	8	45	11	1472	294	$206,534	$123,921
4	6	15	24	4416	883	$619,603	$371,762
4	6	30	12	2208	442	$309,801	$185,881
4	6	45	8	1472	294	$206,534	$123,921
4	7	15	28	5152	1030	$722,870	$433,722
4	7	30	14	2576	515	$361,435	$216,861
4	7	45	9	1717	343	$240,957	$144,574
4	8	15	32	5888	1178	$826,137	$495,682
4	8	30	16	2944	589	$413,068	$247,841
4	8	45	11	1963	393	$275,379	$165,227
5	6	15	24	5520	1104	$774,503	$464,702
5	6	30	12	2760	552	$387,252	$232,351
5	6	45	8	1840	368	$258,168	$154,901
5	7	15	28	6440	1288	$903,587	$542,152
5	7	30	14	3220	644	$451,794	$271,076
5	7	45	9	2147	429	$301,196	$180,717
5	8	15	32	7360	1472	$1,032,671	$619,603
5	8	30	16	3680	736	$516,336	$309,801
5	8	45	11	2453	491	$344,224	$206,534

Step 12: Figure Out What Services You are Going to Offer.

Wholesale labs, meds, imaging, aesthetics, weight loss, OMT, home visits, supplements, in-house pharmacy, fascial distortion work, in house counseling, skin procedures... What and how much can you include in your practice that is mission-consistent for you and adds value for your patients?

Most DPC practices negotiate wholesale pricing on labs and imaging. Some have in-house dispensaries or work with companies that provide cost-transparent medications. There are a whole lot of ways to go about acquiring low prices on services. Here are a few pearls: If the lab bills you directly (called 'client billing') then they have straight forward, no hassle, direct payment. This helps them tremendously. Make payment *easy* for the vendors you want to work with and you can drive prices down.

You will also get lower prices if you go in knowing what kind of pricing other DPC docs are getting. If you explain that you want the lowest possible price because your practice model is to make healthcare accessible and affordable and not to increase your margins while decreasing theirs, you'll get lower pricing. Assure them that you are not dickering their prices down so you can mark them up (if that's honestly what you are going to do). We mark our labs and imaging and medications up 10% or to the nearest dollar (whichever is less). These are not profit sources for us and we never wanted them to be. It's not part of our model. When our lab vendors and imaging companies finally 'got' this, they were willing to lower their rates.

CPT's	Test Name	SPARKmd FEE
80074	Acute Hepatitis Panel (ABC Reflexive)	$45.00
86003 x22	ADULT FOOD PANEL 22	$135.00
87070; 87075; 87205	AEROBIC/ANAEROBIC CULTURE	$27.00
87480; 87510; 87660	Affirm DNA Panel - Trich, BV, Candida	$82.00
86038	ANA	$6.00
86803	ANTI-HCV	$8.00
82310; 84075; 84100; 84550; 85651; 86038; 86060; 86140; 86431	ARTHRITIS PANEL II	$27.00
83520; 86038; 86140; 86160x2; 86225; 86235 x6; 86255; 86431	AUTOIMMUNE PANEL	$70.00
80048	BASIC METABOLIC PANEL	$5.00
84702	B-HCG QUANT	$28.00
83880	B-Type Natriuretic Peptide	$41.00
85025	CBC	$4.00
87491	CHLAMYDIA APTIMA	$28.00
80053	COMPREHENSIVE METABOLIC PANEL	$6.00
86140	C-REACTIVE PROT	$6.00
82550	CREATINE KINASE	$6.00
86141	CRP, Highly Sens	$10.00
85379	D-DIMER	$20.00
87070	DEFINITIVE THROAT CULTURE	$14.00
86225	dsDNA ANTIBODY	$23.00
86665 x2	EPSTEIN-BARR VIRUS PROFILE	$37.00
85651	ESR	$3.00
82670	ESTRADIOL	$10.00
82746	FOLATE	$8.00
84481	FREE T3	$6.00
84439	FREE T4	$5.00
84439; 84443	FREE T4/TSH	$10.00
83001	FSH	$5.00
83001; 83002	FSH AND LH	$10.00
81256; 83891; 83892 x2; 83900; 83909; 83912	HEMOCHROMATOSIS	$111.00
83036	HEMOGLOBIN A1C PANEL	$5.00
87529x2	HERPES SIMPLEX CULTURE	$25.00
86694; 86695; 86696	Herpes Simplex Virus 1 and/or 2 Antibodies, IgG / IgM	$38.00
86703	HIV 1/2	$10.00
87621 x2; 87625	HPV Genotype, 16/18,45	$106.00
87624	HPV, High Risk Type	$57.00
83540	IRON	$5.00
83540; 84466	IRON AND TOTAL IRON BINDING	$4.00
82728; 83540; 84466	IRON DEFICIENCY PANEL	$23.00

83036	HEMOGLOBIN A1C PANEL	$5.00
87529x2	HERPES SIMPLEX CULTURE	$25.00
86694; 86695; 86696	Herpes Simplex Virus 1 and/or 2 Antibodies, IgG / IgM	$38.00
86703	HIV 1/2	$10.00
87621 x2; 87625	HPV Genotype, 16/18,45	$106.00
87624	HPV, High Risk Type	$57.00
83540	IRON	$5.00
83540; 84466	IRON AND TOTAL IRON BINDING	$4.00
82728; 83540; 84466	IRON DEFICIENCY PANEL	$23.00
88305	LEVEL IV SURGICAL PATHOLOGY; GROSS & MICRO EXAM	$65.00
83002	LH	$6.00
80061	LIPID PANEL	$5.00
86617 x2	Lyme Antibodies, IgG / IgM Western Blot	$81.00
82043; 82570	Microalbumin (Creatinine), Random	$11.00
86308	Mononucleosis Screen	$8.00
87491; 87591	N. GONORRHEA AND CHLAMYDIA RNA	$41.00
80100; 80300; 82570; 83986	NIDA DRUG SCREEN (LEGACY LAB)	$41.00
84146	PROLACTIN	$2.00
84153	PSA	$9.00
86431	RHEUMATOID FACTOR	$7.00
89321	Semen count post vasectomy	$6.00
84270	SEX HB GLOBULIN	$13.00
87045; 87046 x3	Stool Culture	$15.00
87177; 87209	Stool Ova and Parasite	$15.00
84480 59	T3 TOTAL	$6.00
84436 59	T4 TOTAL	$5.00
84403	TESTOSTERONE	$10.00
84270; 84403	TESTOSTERONE, FREE + TOTAL	$65.00
99195	THERAPEUTIC PHLEB	$14.00
88175	THINPREP w/ IMAGER (Liquid PAP)	$31.00
86376; 86800	THYROID AUTOANTIBODY GROUP	$16.00
84436; 84443; 84479	THYROID PANEL (HYPO) III	$16.00
84436; 84479	THYROID PANEL I	$12.00
84445	Thyroid Stimulating Immunoglobulin	$89.00
86376	TPO	$15.00
84443	TSH, 3rd GEN.	$5.00
81000; 81001	URINALYSIS	$5.00
81000; 81001	Urinalysis with C&S/Micro if Indicated	$5.00
87088	Urine Culture	$12.00
81003	UROGRAM	$5.00
82607	VITAMIN B12	$7.00
82607; 82746	Vitamin B12 and Folate	$24.00

What about the in-house dispensary (aka pharmacy)?

Some people seem to think it is just too hard or too complicated to have an in-house pharmacy. I find using our autoclave more complicated than running an in house pharmacy. Technically it's called an "in house dispensary". You **must** have an EMR that is designed to manage an in-house pharmacy. For 3 years we used AtlasMD EMR and it ROCKED at this. It managed our whole in-house pharmacy, our dispensing, the inventory, the pricing, the billing... everything.

In house pharmacies are, in my opinion, the cheapest and best marketing you can have for your practice and DPC. Nothing says "we're on the same side" like saving a patient $600/month on their medications right.at.the.point.of.service. Our best win was saving a patient $2100 monthly on ONE medication. And she had insurance. The wins on drug pricing can be unreal.

I have a strong bias which I will openly declare-- If you are in one of the states where you can dispense medications directly to your patients and you would like to do so, you need to buy most if not ALL of your medications from a wholesaler like Andameds. Many generics are about 1/3 the goodrx price if you buy them from Andameds.com or a competitive wholesaler. I would also strongly encourage consideration of AtlasMD EMR. Other solutions include the EMR of your choice partnered with MDScripts or Flexscan for dispensing and the Hint health billing platform.

I'm sure there are other ways to manage dispensing-- in fact there are growing models where you can buy a machine that is loaded with meds and dispenses to patients. Marley Drug is a company on the east coast that will mail low-ish cost medications to patients. And goodrx.com and blink health are two more ways that ANY patient can look at lowest possible cash pricing for meds.

No matter what you decide, you can be flexible and you can change your mind. But the in-house dispensary is just like everything else: a learning curve. Constantly ask yourself: how can I add value? How can I simplify the patient experience and the physician-patient encounter? How can I do better? Your competition, no matter how big, simply cannot meet those needs as fast as an independent, motivated provider can.

In terms of what medications to have on hand/what to order: We have gotten to a point where our pharmacy is pretty 'steady'. The list of our present inventory, at about 550 patients, is included next. I often see docs ask, "What do I have to have in my inventory when I open?" Really, the answer can reasonably be: "Nothing". Build your pharmacy as you build your practice. What's absolutely fantastic about Andameds is that you can place an order and have meds the next day in most locations. Patients don't mind waiting a day or two on meds when they can save money.

Sample drug prices for wholesale drugs (as of 2019)

Name	Generic for	#pills/90 days	90 day supply
Acidophilus		90	$11.16
ACYCLOVIR 400mg/1	Zovirax	270	$19.71
Alendronate 70mg/1	Fosamax	12	$12.94
AMITRIPTYLINE HYDROCHLORIDE 25mg/1	Elavil	90	$20.43
AMLODIPINE BESYLATE 10mg/1	Norvasc	90	$1.26
AMLODIPINE BESYLATE 5mg/1	Norvasc	90	$0.81
AMOXICILLIN; CLAVULANATE POTASSIUM 875mg/1; 125mg/1	Augmentin	20	$6.06
AMOXICILLIN 250mg/5mL - 100 mL in 1 BOTTLE (0143-9889-01)	Amoxil	1	$1.98
AMOXICILLIN 400mg/5mL - 100 mL in 1 BOTTLE (0143-9887-01)	Amoxil	1	$2.18
AMOXICILLIN 500mg/1	Amoxil	30	$1.53
AMOXICILLIN 875mg/1	Amoxil	20	$2.32
Aplisol (Tuberculin Purified Protein Derivative) 5[iU]/.1mL		1	$8.12
ARIPIPRAZOLE 5mg/1	Abilify	90	$69.39
ATENOLOL 100mg/1	Tenormin	90	$2.70
ATENOLOL 50mg/1	Tenormin	90	$1.71
ATORVASTATIN CALCIUM 10mg/1	Lipitor	90	$5.85
ATORVASTATIN CALCIUM 20mg/1	Lipitor	90	$8.19
ATORVASTATIN CALCIUM 40mg/1	Lipitor	90	$9.18
Aviane		3	$28.64
AZELASTINE HYDROCHLORIDE 137ug/1	Astelin	3	$46.48
AZITHROMYCIN MONOHYDRATE 250mg/1	Z-Pack	1	$1.53
Azithromycin 200mg/5mL - 30 mL in 1 BOTTLE (0093-2026-31)	Zithromax susp	1	$13.76
BENAZEPRIL HYDROCHLORIDE 20mg/1	Lotensin	90	$4.59
BENAZEPRIL HYDROCHLORIDE 40mg/1	Lotensin	90	$4.86
BENZONATATE 100mg/1	Tessalon Perles	30	$5.31
Boxer splint, medium right		1	$20.00
BUPROPION HYDROCHLORIDE 150mg/1	Wellbutrin SR	90	$11.07
BUPROPION HYDROCHLORIDE 150mg/1	Wellbutrin	90	$32.94
BUPROPION HYDROCHLORIDE 150mg/1	Wellbutrin XL	90	$32.94
BUPROPION HYDROCHLORIDE 300mg/1	Wellbutrin XL	90	$40.41
CEFTRIAXONE 1g/1 - 10 INJECTION, POWDER, FOR SOLUTION in 1	Rocephin	1	$1.98
CELECOXIB 100mg/1	Celebrex	180	$82.44
CELECOXIB 200mg/1	Celebrex	90	$31.95
CEPHALEXIN 500mg/1	Keflex	21	$1.64
ciprofloxacin 250mg/1	Cipro	20	$2.20
ciprofloxacin 500mg/1	Cipro	20	$2.28
Citalopram 10mg/1	Celexa	90	$1.80
Citalopram 20mg/1	Celexa	90	$1.62
Citalopram 40mg/1	Celexa	90	$2.88
CLONIDINE HYDROCHLORIDE 0.1mg/1	Catapres	270	$4.59
Clopidogrel 75mg/1	Plavix	90	$5.85
CLOTRIMAZOLE; BETAMETHASONE DIPROPIONATE 10mg/g; 0.5mg.	Lotrisone	1	$10.45
CLOTRIMAZOLE 1g/100g - 1 TUBE in 1 CARTON (45802-434-11) > 28	Lotrimin	1	$1.86
Constulose 10g/15mL - 946 mL in 1 BOTTLE (45963-439-65)	Chronulac syrup	1	$11.68
CYANOCOBALAMIN 1000ug/mL	Vitamin B 12	1	$6.08
CYCLOBENZAPRINE HYDROCHLORIDE 10mg/1	Flexeril	90	$2.25
DESOGESTREL AND ETHINYL ESTRADIOL AND ETHINYL ESTRADIO	Mircette	3	$42.84

Drug	Brand	Qty	Price
DICLOFENAC SODIUM 75mg/1	Voltaren	180	$22.86
DICYCLOMINE HYDROCHLORIDE 20mg/1	Bentyl	270	$17.82
DORZOLAMIDE HYDROCHLORIDE 20mg/mL - 1 BOTTLE in 1 CARTON (50383-232-10) > 10		30	$250.47
Doxazosin 4mg/1	Cardura	90	$20.70
Do.			$31.41
Doxycycline Monohydrate (Doxycycline) 50mg/1	Monodox	90	$24.93
DULOXETINE 30mg/1	Cymbalta	90	$25.29
Duloxetine 60mg/1	Cymbalta	90	$27.90
Emily McDowell Cards		1	$3.00
EPINEPHRINE 0.3mg/.3mL	Epipen AUTO INJ	1	$165.00
EPINEPHRINE 1mg/mL - 25 AMPULE in 1 CARTON (0409-7241-01) > 1	Adrenalin	1	$2.56
Escitalopram 10mg/1	Lexapro	90	$4.86
Escitalopram 20mg/1	Lexapro	90	$4.86
Escitalopram 5mg/1	Lexapro	90	$5.31
Estradiol Transdermal System (Estradiol) 0.025mg/d	Climara	1	$58.08
ESTRADIOL 0.5mg/1	Estrace	90	$10.71
ESTRADIOL 1mg/1	Estrace	90	$13.14
ESTRADIOL 2mg/1	Estrace	90	$16.20
FINASTERIDE 5mg/1	Proscar	90	$14.40
FLUCONAZOLE 150mg/1	Diflucan	2	$1.53
Fluoxetine 20mg/1	Prozac	90	$1.80
Fluoxetine 40mg/1	Prozac	90	$8.01
FLUTICASONE PROPIONATE 50ug/1	Flonase	1	$5.48
FUROSEMIDE 40mg/1	Lasix	90	$0.90
GABAPENTIN 100mg/1	Gabapentin	270	$8.10
GEMFIBROZIL 600mg/1	Lipid	90	$12.42
GLIMEPIRIDE 1mg/1	Amaryl	90	$5.49
GLIMEPIRIDE 2mg/1	Amaryl	90	$7.02
HYDROCHLOROTHIAZIDE 25mg/1	Hydrodiuril	90	$0.81
HYDROCHLOROTHIAZIDE 50mg/1		90	$2.79
HYDROXYZINE HYDROCHLORIDE 50mg/1	Atarax	90	$8.46
Junel 1/20 (norethindrone acetate and ethinyl estradiol) 1mg/1; 20ug/1	Loestrin	3	$40.27
Junel Fe 1/20	Loestrin Fe 1.0/20	3	$29.87
KENALOG-40 (TRIAMCINOLONE ACETONIDE) 40mg/mL		1	$9.90
LAMOTRIGINE 100mg/1	Lamictal	90	$3.60
LAMOTRIGINE 25mg/1	Lamictal	90	$4.23
LEVETIRACETAM 750mg/1	Keppra	180	$28.08
LEVOFLOXACIN 500mg/1	Levaquin	10	$2.34
LEVOFLOXACIN 750mg/1	Levaquin	10	$3.10
LISINOPRIL; HYDROCHLOROTHIAZIDE 10mg/1; 12.5mg/1	Zestoretic	90	$2.70
Lisinopril and Hydrochlorothiazide 20mg/1; 12.5mg/1	Zestoretic	90	$2.52
Lisinopril and Hydrochlorothiazide 20mg/1; 25mg/1	Zestoretic	90	$2.88
LISINOPRIL 10mg/1		90	$0.99
LISINOPRIL 20mg/1	Zestril	90	$1.89
LISINOPRIL 40mg/1	Zestril	90	$3.96
LISINOPRIL 5mg/1	Zestril	90	$1.17
LOSARTAN POTASSIUM 100mg/1	Cozaar	90	$4.77
LOSARTAN POTASSIUM 25mg/1	Cozaar	90	$2.52
LOSARTAN POTASSIUM 50mg/1	Cozaar	90	$4.95
LOVASTATIN 20mg/1	Mevacor	90	$9.27
LOVASTATIN 40mg/1	Mevacor	90	$6.57
Major LubriFresh PM (Mineral oil and White petrolatum) 150mg/g; 830m(	Lubrifresh PM	1	$2.72

LOSARTAN POTASSIUM 25mg/1	Cozaar	90	$2.52
LOSARTAN POTASSIUM 50mg/1	Cozaar	90	$4.95
LOVASTATIN 20mg/1	Mevacor	90	$9.27
LOVASTATIN 40mg/1	Mevacor	90	$6.57
Major LubriFresh PM (Mineral oil and White petrolatum) 150mg/g; 830mg	Lubrifresh PM	1	$2.72
MEC			7.98
MELOXICAM 15mg/1	Mobic	90	$1.62
METFORMIN HYDROCHLORIDE ER 500mg/1	Glucophage XR	270	$11.07
METFORMIN HYDROCHLORIDE 500mg/1	Glocophage	360	$4.32
METOPROLOL SUCCINATE 100mg/1	Toprol	90	$35.19
METOPROLOL SUCCINATE 25mg/1	Toprol XL	90	$14.85
METOPROLOL SUCCINATE 50mg/1	Toprol XL	90	$16.56
METOPROLOL TARTRATE 25mg/1	Lopressor	180	$3.42
METOPROLOL TARTRATE 50mg/1	Lopressor	180	$3.78
Metronidazole Topical Gel 7.5mg/g - 1 TUBE in 1 CARTON (66993-962-	Metrogel	1	$65.97
METRONIDAZOLE 500mg/1	Flagyl	21	$7.33
MINOCYCLINE HYDROCHLORIDE 100mg/1	Minocin	90	$59.58
MIRTAZAPINE 15mg/1	Remeron	90	$7.56
MONTELUKAST SODIUM 10mg/1	Singulair	90	$6.66
MUPIROCIN 20mg/g - 22 g in 1 TUBE (68462-180-22)	Bactroban Ointment	1	$5.24
Naproxen Sodium		1	$3.44
Next Choice One Dose (Levonorgestrel) 1.5mg/1	Plan B	1	$26.52
NP Thyroid 60 38ug/1; 9ug/1	Armour Thyroid	90	$40.68
NP Thyroid 90 57ug/1; 13.5ug/1	Armour Thyroid	90	$59.40
NUVARING		1	$0.00
OLANZAPINE 10mg/1	Zyprexa	90	$12.87
OLANZAPINE 15mg/1	Zyprexa	90	$21.51
OLANZAPINE 20mg/1	Zyprexa	90	$29.70
OMEPRAZOLE 20mg/1	Prilosec	90	$5.22
OMEPRAZOLE 40mg/1	Prilosec	90	$5.31
ondansetron 4mg/1	Zofran	30	$4.62
ondansetron 8mg/1	Zofran	30	$8.16
Orthotic support		1	$30.00
OXYBUTYNIN CHLORIDE 5mg/1	Ditropan	180	$61.20
OXYBUTYNIN CHLORIDE 5mg/1	Ditropan XL	90	$49.77
Padded metacarpal splint, left large		1	$20.00
PANTOPRAZOLE SODIUM 40mg/1	Protonix	90	$5.94
Paroxetine 20mg/1	Paxil	90	$6.30
Patella Knee Support Extra Large		1	$10.00
Patella knee support, large		1	$10.00
Patella knee support, medium		1	$10.00
PIOGLITAZONE HYDROCHLORIDE 15mg/1	Acts	90	$11.25
Portia		3	$45.65
POTASSIUM CHLORIDE 20meq	K-Dur	90	$21.78
PREDNISONE 10mg/1	Prednisone	30	$3.33
PREDNISONE 20mg/1		30	$3.90
PROMETHAZINE HYDROCHLORIDE 25mg/1	Phenergan	90	$5.04
QUETIAPINE FUMARATE 25mg/1	Seroquel	90	$4.32
QUETIAPINE FUMARATE 50mg/1	Seroquel	90	$4.50
RIZATRIPTAN BENZOATE 10mg/1	Maxalt	1	$13.97
RIZATRIPTAN BENZOATE 5mg/1	Maxalt	1	$11.78
ROSUVASTATIN CALCIUM 20mg/1	Crestor	90	$15.93

ROSUVASTATIN CALCIUM 20mg/1	Crestor	90	$15.93
SERTRALINE HYDROCHLORIDE 100mg/1	Zoloft	90	$3.78
SERTRALINE HYDROCHLORIDE 25mg/1	Zoloft	90	$3.87
SERTRALINE HYDROCHLORIDE 50mg/1	Zoloft	90	$3.33
Sildenafil 20mg/1		60	$15.06
SIMVASTATIN 10mg/1	Zocor	90	$1.98
SIMVASTATIN 20mg/1	Zocor	90	$1.62
SIMVASTATIN 40mg/1	Zocor	90	$3.24
Spacer		1	$9.46
SPIRONOLACTONE 100mg/1	Aldactone	90	$27.90
SPIRONOLACTONE 25mg/1	Aldactone	90	$5.04
SPIRONOLACTONE 50mg/1		90	$18.81
Sprintec (Norgestimate and Ethinyl Estradiol)		3	$19.86
Stabilizing Ankle Support, Large		1	$15.00
Stabilizing Ankle Support, M		1	$15.00
SULFAMETHOXAZOLE; TRIMETHOPRIM 800mg/1; 160mg/1	Bactrim DS	20	$1.24
SUMATRIPTAN SUCCINATE 100mg/1	Imitrex	1	$6.92
Surround Air Ankle, Regular 10 inch, Left		1	$19.00
Surround Gel Ankle, Regular 10 inch		1	$19.00
T-Shirt (sparkMD)		1	$15.00
TERBINAFINE HYDROCHLORIDE 250mg/1	Lamisil	60	$7.26
Tetanus and Diphtheria Toxoids Adsorbed 2[Lf]/.5mL; 2[Lf]/.5mL	TD	1	$23.10
TOPIRAMATE 25mg/1	Topamax	90	$2.25
TORSEMIDE 20mg/1	Demadex	90	$6.75
TRAZODONE HYDROCHLORIDE 100mg/1	Desyrel	90	$8.82
TRAZODONE HYDROCHLORIDE 50mg/1	Desyrel	90	$4.05
TRIAMCINOLONE ACETONIDE 1mg/g - 1 TUBE in 1 CARTON (0713-0228-15) > 15 g in 1 TUE		1	$2.64
TRIAMCINOLONE ACETONIDE 5mg/g - 15 g in 1 TUBE (67877-318-15	Kenalog	1	$5.84
TRIAMTERENE; HYDROCHLOROTHIAZIDE 25mg/1; 37.5mg/1	Maxzide	90	$13.41
TRIAMTERENE; HYDROCHLOROTHIAZIDE 75mg/1; 50mg/1	Maxzide	90	$13.68
Vagifem (estradiol) 10ug/1		8	$0.00
VALACYCLOVIR HYDROCHLORIDE 1g/1	Valtrex	4	$1.90
VENLAFAXINE HYDROCHLORIDE 75mg/1	Effexor	90	$11.16
VENTOLIN HFA (albuterol sulfate) 90ug/1 - 1 INHALER in 1 CARTON (0	Ventolin	1	$22.88
VERAPAMIL HYDROCHLORIDE 180mg/1	Isoptin ER	90	$11.61
VITAMIN D (ergocalciferol) 1.25I/1		8	$0.86
Wrist Support Large Left		1	$7.00
Wrist Support Large Right		1	$7.00
Wrist Support Medium Left		1	$7.00
Wrist Support Medium Right		1	$7.00
Wrist Support Small Left		1	$7.00
Wrist Support Small Right		1	$7.00

Step 13: Write Your Business Plan.

Business plans have an accepted format, just like a living will or your first SOAP note. You can download templates online. Our first business plan took me two months from 10pm – 2am to write, was thirty-three glorious pages, was probably overkill but it got the job done. We modified a downloadable template from entrepreneur.com. And then we worked on it (a lot). In the end, it was and has been a very powerful tool for us to understand and market our business and was the tool that helped us get loans to start sparkMD and buy a building.

There are a number of ways to get help with your business plan and your business vision. SCORE is the "Service Core of Retired Executives" and is a group of, you guessed it, retired executives who have a lot of business experience and provide free business consultation in most communities. SBA.gov is the government sponsored site for small business and has an incredible amount of resources and data. We've mentioned BNI. And think about utilizing your local community college or university for resources for free marketing plans and for help with entrepreneurship. (One idea: approach a marketing professor before the year starts to see if they want to use you as a 'project').

A side note on the 'promise' of your brand. From your vision you get your mission statement- the verbose version of your promise. As you simplify this statement, you get your promise. Then from your simplified promise you have your slogan. And from your slogan, you can make your brand. When you know your brand, the name and logo come (somewhat) easily.

Step 14: Bricks & Mortar: Floorplans & Design.

Whether you buy or lease you're going to need to sort out a floor plan and choose paint colors, carpet, flooring, decor. It's possible to do all of this on a budget. Pinterest helps, as does eBay, TJMaxx, Craigslist and elbow grease.

You need to find out what the requirements are for you to have a small outpatient medical clinic. Buildings are zoned for various purposes. You probably have a planning & zoning office in your community. Call them and find out what type of zoning requirements exist for outpatient primary care medical office space. You may have to explain, repeatedly, that you don't do sedation, or surgery, or have chemical fumes (like a salon). The more broad your zoning, the more options available to you and the lower your lease price.

Most businesses also need an 'operating license'. In Idaho (and in most states), having an active state license to practice medicine is your 'operating license'. You might need to discuss this with planning & zoning or your local medical board for clarification.

Typically in commercial real estate the landlord pays for the build-out (renovation) of the space for the tenant, although not always. It's also quite customary for tenants to negotiate a few months of no lease- particularly if it's during the build out or first few months of a new business. Don't be afraid to negotiate for what you need.

Commercial real estate is billed on a square foot/year pricing structure, often with a "triple N"-or triple net lease. According to Wikipedia: "A triple net lease (triple-Net or NNN) is a lease agreement on a property where the tenant or lessee agrees to pay all real estate taxes, building insurance, and maintenance (the three "nets") on the property in addition to any normal fees that are expected under the agreement (rent, utilities, etc.)." Depending on the property, pricing of a lease plus NNN can get spendy. Map it all out and ask a lot of questions. Make sure you know how the lease pricing changes from one year to the next and what the options for lease extension and departure are. Having a commercial real estate agent who gets what you are wanting to do is invaluable for this process.

A side note on commercial real estate agents-- in our experience this is an interesting group of professionals. They don't seem to get much business/work in the wintertime (Nov-January). They are looking for the next big mega-mall. Little deals (like a family doc wanting to buy a modest space for a low cost medical clinic) are not appealing to most commercial agents. We interviewed 6 (six!) agents- before we found an agent who was inspired, understood what we were wanting to do and who was on-board to help us. Don't give up and don't let your business vision be compromised by inflated real-estate pricing. Be firm, negotiate and don't be afraid to walk away if you must. And get EVERYTHING (every.thing.) in writing. Everything.

DPC doctors operate out of anywhere from a single 200 sq foot room with shared reception space all the way to a 3000 square foot (or more) clinic with lab, X-Ray room, DEXA scanner, space for cosmetic treatments & massage, etc... Your size is going to depend on your vision now, in the future and what kind of resources you have.

In residency I 'needed' 4 rooms operational for the nurses to stay ahead of me. In DPC, I need 1 room. Occasionally, if I'm running late, or as we grow, it's nice to have 2 rooms, but a 1:1 ratio of providers to exam rooms seems to work for most people.

Our floor plan is attached. We love our clinic. Love! It is open and bright and does NOT feel like a dreary medical place. There are a few thing we would change, though:

1. We would add in many, many more electrical outlets. Decide what you need and double it.
2. Consider putting your doors on the wall 'past' the room. Consider what you can see when you open the doors. In our main exam room (the second one) there is a clear line of sight from the waiting room into the room to the exam table. We hung long IKEA curtains as a solution.
3. You can make it TOO inviting. Use visual cues as 'barriers' so people don't just wander on back into your office
4. Have a door on your office.
5. If you have a lab draw station, have it near the front of the clinic.
6. Set up your nurses/front desk with safety in mind. We should have put our entry desk on the opposite wall so that if there was an emergency or problem patient our staff could get out the side door without having to walk around the desk and through the hall. (We installed a panic button, instead).
7. Put in GOOD toilets.

8. We love our big doors. We have no issues navigating wheelchairs and have had more visits from the paramedics than we would like and everyone can navigate the space easily
9. You don't need a big break room.
10. If your vision is to go and add providers, and you have the space, AND your spouse is part of the business vision, consider a space that can be a private office for you as the owner.
11. And last, but not least, try to leave room to grow. You will move and rearrange and adjust as you grow. It's just part of the business model.

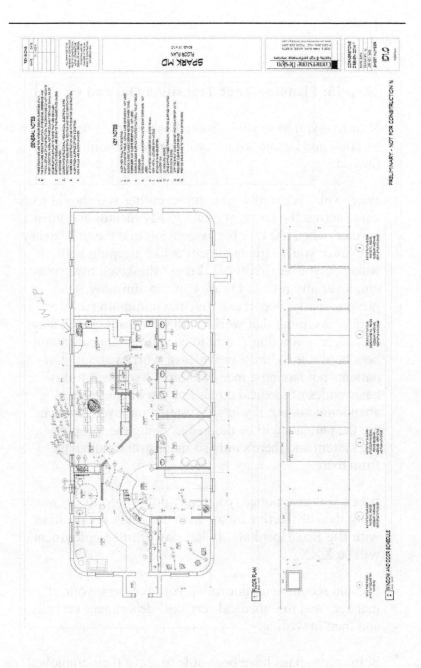

Cornerstone Design

SPARK MD
FLOOR PLAN

PRELIMINARY - NOT FOR CONSTRUCTION %

Step 15: Planning Your Transition Out and In.

Now that you have your vision, business plan, logo, location and business name you can really solidify your timeline.

When you reviewed your contract earlier you should have come across the terms of quitting. My mentor and former partner, when she quit her system job told me that "every day (after you've given notice) is like sleeping with someone you've divorced." I don't think you owe your employer any favors. I think you can amicably, professionally, depart and give the minimum required notice, assuming that works with your plans. Don't stay on longer if you don't want to because of appeals about how hard it is to hire a provider or worries about your patients not having a medical home. You must follow basic codes of medical ethics and laws about patient abandonment, but if you are system employed, chances are the patients will be defined as being the 'property' of the system and there's only so much you can manage from there.

When you give notice, you really don't need to say much more than "Effective today, I am resigning my position with Big Box Hospital. My last day of full employment will be XXX."

I would recommend informing your partners, your office manager and the 'medical services' department verbally and then in writing.

Some physicians have been able to leave their employed job with the full support of their employer. If this is your situation, get ready! You can build your DPC beginnings while you're still getting paid by the system.

Town Halls!

A number of DPC docs who were able to discuss their practice transition have had very good success with town halls and progressive direct marketing to interested patients and small businesses. Dr. Kissi Blackwell of Clarity Direct Health Care in Wichita Falls, Texas and Dr. Jennifer Harader at Oasis Family Medicine in Topeka, Kansas shared their very successful (and similar) paths to growth and starting with income.

I also was able to solicit my patients. I had a non-compete and non-solicitation clause in my employment contract but I had a very good working relationship with our hospital CEO. I asked him to waive both and, after reassurance that I was not going to work for the competitor, he did so. (I think this is a good point about how we don't have to get immediately litigious about everything.) Once my resignation was public (around November 2014), I started explaining what I was going to be doing to any patients that I wanted to recruit and that showed the slightest interest.

My last day as an employed doc was 12/24/2014. I spent Christmas day stuffing envelopes and sent out about 300-400 letters introducing the new practice and directing them to our website and Facebook page. (This covered around 1000 patients due to sending them to households). Our website went live 12/31 and pre-enrollment began. I didn't open until 3/2/2015 so during that 3 months I met with anyone in the business community that was willing to sit down with me. We hosted 2 town hall meetings for small businesses and 1 for individuals. They were relativity poorly attended (max of 30 ppl), but they served the purpose of planting seeds. A few people signed up right away as a result, but most of the fruit from those was delayed or came from our attendees telling others about the practice. I ended up opening with ~250 pre-enrollments. Most of those were prior patients of mine, but that group now comprises only 1/3 of my panel.

I was very lucky in that I was able to solicit my patients. I would also talk to whoever would listen. I had to get out of my comfort zone in that sense bc I'm normally a very quiet person. I talked to several local business owners while I was eating out or having coffee. Some of them let me leave cards or post my flyer at their establishment. Having the website ready right off the bat was so helpful bc when I didn't have much time to explain, I could direct them there and that helped me get emails in order to do more directed marketing. I started sending out a newsletter to all the people that signed up on my website and that was part of how I marketed my Town Hall. I also was able to send a letter out to all my patients with details about my town hall and my contact info. I got a Google Voice number and started answering all the calls myself. It was exhausting to talk to each individual myself but I'm still doing it and that is what seems to be working best. I feel like they have to hear it from the horse's mouth. My nurse would try to explain or my sister (she works at the hospital) but until the spoke w me, it did not click. One other thing I feel is super important and something one of the other docs told me a year ago.... start acting like a DPC doc NOW. Answer your own phone calls as much as you can, give a select few you cell phone. I ended up with an amazing article in the paper bc my patient wrote it. A week before, he started having an issue with his BP. He messaged me on Twitter and I began changing his meds and asking him to send me his readings at different times of the day. I fixed his BP in real time and he as so impressed, he said that made up his mind about whether to sign up and he wrote the best article!

So, figure out your contract. Plan that on the day your departure is public- if you are allowed- to begin telling everyone who will listen about what you are doing. Your days will be long. Have a flash page or functional website where you can direct people to learn more. Have business cards (even if they're quick ones from vistaprint) and carry them around to give to people who want to find you/learn more. Build an email list of interested people and invite them to informational town halls before you open. Take pre-enrollment payment information and set it up to begin billing the day you open.

Other considerations before you leave your employed job: work with HR (once your departure is known) to figure out options for life insurance, disability insurance, 401K/403b roll-overs and continuation of health insurance. If you can get all of these things in place while you have a substantial income, you will have a better benefit.

Get a copy of all of your prior malpractice coverage certificates from your employer.

Notify insurance companies that you are no longer participating with them OR try to get in writing from your employer that they will address that matter.

Should you opt out of Medicare?

Around the time you give notice (usually 3-4 months are required) you are about four to six months away from opening your DPC practice. It's time to decide if you are going to opt-out of Medicare and to solidify any side-jobs, if you intend to have one.

There are two resources I would recommend in your decision making and transition to opt out of Medicare. The AAPS (http://aapsonline.org/opting-out-of-medicare-a-guide-for-physicians/) and, www.dpcfrontier.com. Phil Eskew has done such a superb job with explaining the ins and outs of the legal side of Medicare opt-out status that I am not going to repeat it here. Your timeline for opting out should be *at least* two months before your desired opt-out date. The schedule of how all of this happens is a bit weird, so plan ahead.

Step 16: Bricks & Mortar: Getting the Goods.

Now you're closing in on opening! It's time to get in the weeds and pick out your clinic resources and start negotiating lab and imaging agreements.

First things first- get a business credit card (while you still have a system job). We have the Spark Visa from Chase. The Spark name is a coincidence. It has served us well and is one of the higher rated business credit cards. You can find reviews of business credit cards online and apply. Here's one source: https://www.nerdwallet.com/blog/top-credit-cards/nerdwallets-best-small-business-credit-cards/

Time to pick an EMR.

You do not HAVE to have an EMR. Paper, a word document or any other solution that's sensible to you and privacy secured will work. Some of these solutions aren't scalable, but they'll work. EMR's that are popular in DPC include atlasMD, Elation, Cerbo, amazingcharts/InLight, soapware, eMD, MD-HQ, Athena, and Practicefusion. If you join any of the many Facebook forums on DPC, there's ample information about what docs think of these tools.

Set up supplier relationships. There is a list of suppliers at the end of this document in the resources section. We use Andameds (it takes a few weeks to get your account going and get your first order in), Costco, Amazon and Moore Medical, now merged with McKesson. We've ordered from Henry Schein once in 3 years. Those are our vendors. There are innumerable others, however, that work for many DPC docs.

Meet with lab companies and imaging centers. Transparent pricing (knowing what prices other doctors are getting) and explaining your model will help you drive down pricing. Bring other doctors pricing lists in when you negotiate. Get the best rates you can and then renegotiate yearly to drive prices down further.

Step 17: Time to Market Your Practice!

One DPC question is, "how do you effectively market DPC?"

It's valuable to ask what this means. In the marketing world this is measured by return on investment. For every dollar spent, how many dollars are made. This amount varies widely by industry.

In my opinion, because of the very low cost of DPC, most forms of traditional marketing simply don't make sense. If a newspaper ad costs $800 to run for 1 week, and you get one loyal customer from it, it is just *barely* worth the expense. $800 spent on Facebook advertising would last more than 3 months and generate tens, if not hundreds of thousands of clicks and views.

The marketing that has seemed to work for many DPC docs is

Pound the pavement. Get out there. Set 'communication goals'. Talk to anyone who will listen. Figure out how to meet with and communicate with small business owners. Show them how you can help their business grow.

Know your elevator pitch. This is the 20-30 second, high level overview of what you do. Our pitch is basically: "At sparkMD we are a low-cost, cash-based outpatient medical clinic. We provide same and next day visits, visits by phone and email, home visits and hospital visits to our patient members for less than $3/day. Healthcare doesn't have to be expensive, or unpleasant. We can save most people, whether they have insurance or not, up to

80% on their healthcare spend." If people are really interested this is where I usually tell a specific story about cost savings or access or weekend phone triage that saved a specific patient hassle, time and money.

Have town halls (this has been discussed but it is very good marketing).

Set up a business Facebook page and post frequently. Boost successful posts for $5-$10 dollars to extend your reach.

Make your website work for you. You can build your own website via wix.com, weebly or wordpress.com but if you are not saavy hire someone to build a functional site and to optimize your search engine functionality. A nice starter website can be done for < $3000.

Other places to get out and speak include BNI, your local business chamber and church groups. Or send targeted letters to twenty small businesses within five to ten miles of your clinic. Follow the letter with a phone call.

Radio ads are less expensive than newspaper which are less expensive than TV and, in my opinion, none of them have a high enough ROI to justify their cost, especially in the beginning.

There are a lot of ways to build your business and you don't have to spend a lot of money, particularly if you're willing to do the work. Alternatively, if you have a ton of money laying around, I suppose you could hire a marketing firm and do TV, radio and print ads and let the rest of us know if it works!

Step 18. Protect Yourself: Making it All Legit.

DPC presents an interesting challenge; you must be able to tolerate enough risk to be entrepreneurial but you also have to know when the rules still apply to you. To complicate matters: a number of laws around how you practice, how you dispense meds, and work-force related laws vary by state.

Read dpcfrontier for the most up to date legal matters in DPC.

Get a mentor in your home state, if you can, to help with what road blocks he or she ran into before opening.

Briefly:

Do you know if your state has a law for DPC? You should. Check **www.dpcfrontier.com**

Do you know if you can dispense medications in your state?

Do you have a patient contract? (Phil has a great 'template' and ours is attached at the end-- it's a modification of Phil's work).

Here's a few of the 'hot' topics in DPC and legal matters:

HIPAA, in its most strict interpretation, applies to the electronic transmission of patient information. It comes up: does HIPAA apply to DPC? I suppose, technically, If you are not electronically transmitting *anything ever* then HIPAA doesn't apply to you. But this really is the minutiae of HIPAA and the spirit of patient privacy matters. Most DPC docs have their patients sign a privacy agreement and have disclaimers on the limits of privacy with electronic communication. This is an area where, again, I would defer to Phil Eskew. Bare bones, HIPAA is: a patient privacy agreement, a communication disclaimer on all electronically transmitted communication, a staff privacy document (for when you hire people) and a once a year review of what you are doing to keep patient information secure. This doesn't have to be a one week project. There are open source HIPAA training and compliance resources on-line that are useful and meet this very basic practice standard. Don't make things difficult just because you can or just because that's how things were done in your last job. Your trying to transform the broken system, right? So transform it.

HSAs--Oh.My.Goodness. Let me just start by saying that this is a hotly fought, many times debated issue. As of 2020 there remains incredible disagreement about the utilization of HSA's in a DPC setting. The IRS has clearly stated it is illegal to use and, most likely to even FUND an HSA if you are paying a medical practice on a membership basis. Does this make sense? No. Do I like it? No. But please, please, please *listen* and understand that until FEDERAL TAX legislation passes that forces the IRS to change their take on membership-based practices, using HSA for a periodic fee is not legal. Will anything happen to your patients if they pay you this way? Probably not. But can you be sure of that? No. And I don't comment on anything related to the IRS with my patients because I'm not an IRS expert.

Patients CAN use their HSAs to pay for fee-for-service care and for things like imaging, labs and medications. But again, theoretically, funding an HSA while paying a periodic membership fee is seen by the IRS as having 'dual' health plans. It is my sincere hope that this will change very soon, but that is the status of affairs from 2014-2020 thus far.

Much legislation and a President's Executive Order have been put forward to solve this challenge and clear up IRS law so that people can clearly fund an HSA, and use those funds to pay their doctor directly.. The Primary Care Enhancement Act was introduced in 2016-2017 and revised and revised and revised. Organizations such as The Direct Primary Care Coalition, The DPC Alliance and DPCAction are three very different places to obtain information about the present state of politics, legislation and DPC. Please be mindful that each organization has it's own mission and purpose so the information from each will differ. (I have served on the Board for the DPC Coalition and am President 2020-2021 of the DPC Alliance so present this information but have clear personal biases). Above all, be informed. And do your best to inform yourself across multiple platforms. At times information has been shared through Facebook groups and is not always 100% correct.

CLIA- Even if you do the simplest thing (like a rapid strep swab) you need a CLIA waiver. Google "CLIA waiver for medical clinic", download the form, fill it out and send it in. Note: if you want to do anything with a microscope there is a special part for that. It might take 3-4 months for your first waiver to come through so plan for that.

OSHA and Employment law- Different states have different employment laws. Depending on your risk tolerance and your state laws you may just need a poster informing your staff of their rights to be OSHA compliant or you may need much more. Medtrainer.com charges a monthly fee and many DPC practices state it helps them feel confident about OSHA and employment law.

Dr. Kimberly Corba is a DPC physician who has written a 600+ page comprehensive compliance manual for DPC practices. You can purchase this from her if you desire. I have personally looked through the entire thing and, while some people may find it very helpful, my greatest joy in DPC is unencumbering myself and my practice from as many things as I can. This manual is *not* any legal or procedural standard for DPC. It was borne of a lot of very hard work, legal and business consultation, time and effort. You might find it helpful. Be aware, however, it is far more complex than many believe necessary.

Step 19: Getting to Open.

Oh.my.gosh. You are almost done! In the last three to five weeks you will be very busy. Don't have weekend plans other than to work, move furniture, call patients and make sure things work.

Sign yourself up as a patient and work hard to see both sides of your emails, billing, phones\ and portal. Send out labs on yourself and see how they come back. In the first few months (or years) review ALL of your bills... You'll be shocked how many are incorrect. I think big box clinics hemorrhage money in erroneous billing.

Consider setting up a ribbon cutting with your local Chamber of Commerce. It's great small business marketing.

Begin scheduling patients

Offer to any pre-enrolled patients and to small business friends (such as folks you've met from BNI) to talk to their employees/employers, church groups, friends, etc...

Set aside time every week to work ON the business versus IN the business.

Set one month, three month and six month business goals. Back them out into a task list for your working ON the business time.

As you grow your practice, maintain enough structure with the patient visit to keep it sustainable (don't let every visit be 60 minutes just because you can...-ahem-).

Use your early growth time to set up social media and Facebook posting schedules and sign up for other doctor/healthcare/DPC blogs where you can use other people's education in your blogs.

Now it's time to OPEN!!!

Step 20: Be Hungry!

Now you're open! You did it!!

Show up every day. Take pictures and look back at what you're building. You're going to be tired. You're going to work hard, but for most of us it's really rewarding work.

Build your dream and BELIEVE in it.

Have rules for yourself, your work hours, your staff and your practice and stick to them. Modify as needed, but have rules.

Build networks and friends who are small business owners.

Know that the churn in DPC is very real. Up to 30% of patients who come to you will leave early, come and go or lie or won't pay. Don't take it personally. Keep your eye on your vision, stay positive and move forward. It happened in your other practice, too, you just didn't know it!

And finally, keep a tight watch on the money. Spend on only what you need and get the money flowing as quickly as you can...

You're going to learn a lot as you go. I've said for the last six years... It's like flying down the highway and trying to change the tires on the car. You'll get it done, it's just terrifying!

Acknowledgements

There is so, so, much more to say and so much work to do. This is not a comprehensive DPC tome but hopefully it adds positively to the resources that are presently available. And, hopefully it helps YOU feel inspired to be the doctor you set out to be.

The DPC community is a collaborative community. Thank you to all of my amazing DPC physician colleagues and friends who so readily helped me or inspired me or in any other way informed this document. A particular thanks to Dr. Josh Umbehr, who provided unending and invaluable mentorship in my start-up years, to Dr. Vance Lassey, Dr. Phil Eskew, Dr. Jennifer Harader, Dr Kissi Blackwell and Dr. Nicholas Tomsen, Dr. Douglas Farrago- each provided specific resources or personal input into this project and to my other encouraging, creative, supportive physician friends. Thank you to Kenon Kildew, FNP and Erin Love McDermott, PA-C for the reading and re-readings of this document and for joining me in making sparkMD part of the DPC revolution.

Thanks most of all to my amazing, supportive, hard-working and endlessly patient and loving husband.

And to my girls for reminding me that I am the glitter and daddy is the glue. And together we four do great things.

There's a difference between down-right plagiarism and modifying someone else's work to grow yours. If you use my work, please provide proper credit. For further mentoring, please reach out to the Direct Primary Care Alliance. The online resource "DPCU" is the summation of the work of dozens of DPC physicians and is free.

Never forget the work we do is a privilege. And there are so many of us, wanting to make things better. Now, go be amazing!!

RESOURCES:

Resource 1: Where to Get What and How

DPC sites:
- **www.dpcalliance.org**
- www.dpcfrontier.com
- **www.bagelmd.com**
- www.dpcare.org
- www.atlas.md/starter
- **community.hint.com**

DPC Friendly EMR Vendors:
- AtlasMD EMR
- Elation
- MD-HQ
- Cerbo
- e-clinicalworks
- Athena
- Amazingcharts/InLight
- PracticeFusion
- Soapnotes
- Simple Practice

Billing tools to support cash-based care and membership management:
- AtlasMD EMR
- Hint health
- Twin Oaks
- Square

Tools for inventory management and in-house medication dispensing:
- AtlasMD EMR
- FlexScan
- MD Scripts
- Proficient Rx

Where to get clinical supplies (instruments, chairs, scales, tables)
- Your local hospital's overstock warehouse (really!)
- Amazon
- eBay
- **medsupplier.com**
- Moore Medical (David Drew is my rep and takes more than 30% off published prices).
- Henry Schein
- McKesson
- Most docs have figured out how to be in a GPO.

Where to get medications, injectables, lab supplies, gauze etc:
- Andameds: **www.andameds.com**
- Amazon
- eBay Moore Medical
- Henry Schein
- McKesson
- Advantage Medical Supply (Texas) 210-599-1991
- US Med Source
- **dormer.com**

Cash based surgery options for patients:
- Surgery center of Oklahoma
- St. George Surgery Center
- **affordablehernias.com**

OSHA and labor compliance:
- **medtrainer.com**

Where to purchase websites:
- www.godaddy.com
- for .MD domains:
- Max.md - to purchase .md domains
- **gandi.com** to purchase .md domains

Tools to manage Facebook posts:
- buffer.com

Where to get health insurance:
- ehealthinsurance.com

Where to get low cost meds/medication information:
- iodine.com medication site for patients
- goodrx.com
- Blink health

Marketing/minivideos:
- Sparkol for 90 second videos
- 90secondexplainervideos.com
- thedrawshop.com for drawing marketing
- powtoon

Hearing tests:
- Audiogram mobile app for the iphone with Panasonic RP-HTX7

IUDs:
- www.archpatientassistance.com - for skyla and mirena

Websites:
- Etsy
- Entermotion: www.entermotion.com (out of Wichita)
- www.websmithguy.com

Logos:
- 99designs.com
- www.etsy.com
- www.entermotion.com
- Fiverr.com

Legal help:
- legalzoom.com
- DIY LLC: incfile.com

Medication Disposal
- **medflats.com**
- stericycle.com
- Watch for local med disposal/biohazard collection dates in your community
- Sharps, Inc

Biohazard Disposal
- Stericycle.com
- Sharps, Inc

Online services
- **betterhelp.com** -- online therapists
- talkspace.com

EKG options:
- **alivecor.com**
- **www.smartheartpro.com**

Bluetooth mailboxes:
- **www.perma-vault.com**

Prescription paper:
- Amazon

Sharps Containers:
- Amazon
- Sharps, Inc

Pill bottles:
- Amazon
- Andameds

Business Cards:
- **moo.com**
- **vistaprint.com**
- www.canva.com

Door/Window vinyl signage:
- doityourselflettering.**com**
- **vistaprint.com**
- (Many others)

T-shirts:
- **customink.com**

Cabinets, countertops, appliances, furniture:
- **greendemolitions.com** now called angelrenovations.com (they will negotiate)
- TJMaxx/Homegoods
- Craigslist
- IKEA

Containers/organizers:
- IKEA (particularly IVAR, BESTA and ALGOT systems)
- **containerstore.com** – expensive
- Uline.com (great for pulldown bins for labs)
- Livinbox – on amazon great bins for stacking/pill bottles

Phone Services & Faxing Solutions:
- **ringcentral.com**
- 8x8
- Vontage
- **oooma.com** (virtual assistant)
- GV Mate (google voice mate device)
- **webfones.com**
- Grasshopper
- Faxage.com
- SRFax.com

Online appointment scheduling software:
- Acuity scheduling
- Candarly
- IntakeQ

Floorplanning tool:
- **sketchup.com**
- Floor plans pro:
  http://www.greenteaapps.com/floorplans/

Other mush-mash resources
- Anazao for testosterone?
- Cnect ?
- **MDsave.com**
- **www.docswhocare.com**
- **sharpscompliance.com**
- **www.sba.gov** (small business start up data, advice, business plans).
- **singulairsleep.com** home sleep studies
- Simple**contacts.com** for contact lens renewal
- **warbyparker.com** for cheap glasses
- **www.medicaldevicedepot.com**
- **koleid.com**
- Ynab - accounting software
- Enom

Insurance companies that 'get' DPC
- Allied National

Low cost Pathology:
- Cole Diagnostics

GPOs:
- Premier/Yankee
- Doctorschoice.net

For legal matters: **www.dpcfrontier.com**
and for political matters **dpcare.org**

The start up savings as a member of the DPC Alliance are tremendous. (And I am a founding member so this is biased). Join at dpcalliance.org.

Reference 2: Clinic Lab Inventory at the 2 year mark

COMPANY	PRODUCT	REF #
Quidel	Strep A tests	20122
Quidel	QuickVue In Line Strep A tests	343
Quidel	QuickVue One step hCG Urine test	20109
Siemens	Multistix 10 SG Urine analysis strips	2161
Norco	320 M gloves for nitrogen gas	N/A
Alere BinaxNOW	Influenza A&B cards	416-110
DynRX	Blue Surgical face masks w/ ear loops	2207
Doctor Easy	Rhino ear washer the elephant ear washer bag of 20	
Doctor Easy	Elephant ear washer bottle and sprayer	
Integra	Miltex premium grade instrument brushes	3-1000
Debrox	Earwax removal kit	
Delmar Cenage Learning	Basic Chemical Laboratory Technology sixth edition	
Pyramex	Ztek goggles	S2510S
	5L Grey Soak Buckets	
	7Qt Grey Soak Buckets	
Aqualite System	1000 mL 0.9% Sodium Chloride Irrigation	2099
Aqualite System	1000 mL Sterile Water for Irrigation	3336
Brymill	Cryogun CR-Y AC	
	3Lt 24 hour urine container	
Derma Pak-its	Iodoform packing strip .25"x5yds	59146
firstaid	100 adhesive bandages 0.75"x3"	
Coverlet	2"x2.5" 50 large digits	01307-00

Cypress Medical products	4"x4" gauze sponges 12 ply	
Coverlet	2 1/8" x1.5" 100small digits	01306-00
Coverlet	4"x2.75" 50 patches	78010-00
Careband	Sterile bandages 0.75"x3"	CBD5302
Covidien	Curity Sheer bandage 7/8"	44120
Moore Medical	Fabric Adhesive Bandages Extra Large 2"x4"	68185
Moore Medical	Fabric Adhesive Bandages 1"x3"	68181
Dokal	Wound closure strips 1/8"x3"	5150
Systagenixadaptic	Non-adhering dressing	2012
3M	tegaderm film 2 3/8"x2 3/4"	9505W
3M	tegaderm film 4"x4.75"	9506W
Kendall	Curlty nonadhearing dressing 3"x3"	6112
DermaBlade	Blade to remove skin	72001
Moore Medical	biopsy punch	87052
Healthlink	Biopsy Punch 4.0mm	BP40
Miltex	Stainless Steel Disposable scaples #15	4-415
Redilon	Nonabsorbable surgical suture 45cm	N69931
Ethicon	Ethilon black monofiliment 4-0 18"	699
Ethicon	Ethilon black monofiliment nylon 4-0 18"	69901
GlassVan	Sterile surgical blades#15 No 3	ISO7740
Moore Medical	Surgical Blades #11	3101
	liquid skin	
3M	Precise disposable skin stapler	78-8083-1349-4
Proadvantage	Plain sterile towel drapes 18"x26"	N207100
Proadvantage	cotton dipped applicators	76700
Covidien	Kerlix bandage roll 2.25"x9'	6720

Bovie	high tempature cautery elongated tip	AA21
3M	Coban self-adherent wrap in multiple widths, lengths, and colors	1583
Carefusion	Chloraprep Onestep 1.5mL FREPP	80233
Hibiciens	Antiseptic skin cleanser 16 fluid oz	234057516
PDI	prevantics swabstick 1.6 mL	S40750
Procare	thumbsplint 7" universal	79-92170
Procare	CAS wrist support Sm, Right	79-87153
Procare	CTS wrist support Med, left	79-87165
Procare	CTS wrist support Lg, right	79-81157
Procare	CTS wrist support Lg, left	79-87155
Procare	Knee support w/ patella extra large	79-82638
Welch Allyn	250 thermometer probe covers	65031
Welch Allyn	universal kleenspec single use 2.75mm pediatric specula	52432-U
Welch Allyn	universal kleenspec adult specula 4.25mm	52434-U
Covidien	curity alcohol prep 2ply med	5750
Nitriderm	surgical gloves size 6.5	135650
Nitriderm	surgical gloves size 7.5	135750
Savage Labratories	Surgical Lube	0281-0205-37
Dynarex	white petrolatum	1145
Ansell micro touch nitle	L medical exam gloves	6034513
Sempermed	Med medical exam gloves	TTNF203
Swan	70% Isopropyl Alcohol 1Qt	
Midmark	Speed Clean 16oz	002-0396-00
Integra	Miltex Surgical Instrument Cleaner	3-720

Briston-Myers Squibb	Kenalog-40	
Lopin	ceftriaxone for injection	
Greenstone Brand	Medroxy-progesterone acetate injectable suspension, USP 150 mg/mL	
Hospira Inc.	2% Lidocaine HCl	
Hospira Inc.	8.4% Sodium Bicarbonate USP	
American regent	cyanoco balamin	
Hi-tech	lidocaine 2.5% & prilocaine 2.5% cream	
Hospira Inc.	Ketorolaetromethamine injection	
Mylan	EpiPen 2 pak	
Hospira Inc.	Lidocaine HCl 2% & Epinephrine	
Person & Convey Inc.	Drylsol 35cc	
Fougera	Triple Antibiotic ointment	
Watson	Ipratropium bromide & Albuterol sulfate Inhalation solution	
Rutter by Midmark	M9D AutoClave Sterilizer	
Drucker Co.	Horizon model 642B Centrifuge	
Covidien	Sharps Safey box	
BD	assorted 3,5, 10mL syringes & needles (18g, 23g, 25g, 27g)	

Reference 3: Sample Patient Contract

DIRECT PRIMARY CARE PATIENT AGREEMENT
PRACTICE, LLC

This is an Agreement between PRACTICE NAME (**Practice**), a STATE NAME located at LEGAL PRACTICE ADDRESS, PHYSICIAN NAME, MD (**Physician**) in her/his capacity as an agent of PRACTICE NAME, LLC and You (**Patient**).

Background
The Physician practices family medicine and delivers care on behalf of PRACTICE NAME, LLC in PRACTICE CITY AND STATE. In exchange for certain fees paid by Patient, Practice, through its Physician, agrees to provide Patient with the Services described in this Agreement on the terms and conditions set forth in this Agreement. The practice website is https://www.PRACTICE.com.

Definitions
1. Patient. Patient is defined as those persons for whom Physician shall provide Services, and who are signatories to and incorporated by reference to this agreement.

2. Services. As used in this Agreement, the term Services shall mean a package of ongoing primary care services, both medical and non-medical and certain amenities (collectively **Services**), which are offered by Practice, and set forth in Appendix 1. Patient will be provided with methods to contact the physician via phone, email, and other methods of electronic communication. Physician will make every effort to address the needs of the Patient in a timely manner, but cannot guarantee availability, and cannot guarantee that the patient will not need to seek treatment in the urgent care or emergency department setting.

3. Fees. In exchange for the services described herein, Patient agrees to pay Practice the amount as set forth in Appendix 1, attached. Applicable enrollment fees are payable upon execution of this agreement. These fees may change with time. Patient will be notified 30 days in advance of any fee changes.

4. Non-Participation in Insurance. Patient acknowledges that neither Practice, nor Physician, participate in any health insurance or HMO plans. Dr. PHYSICIAN has opted-out of Medicare. Patient acknowledges that federal regulations REQUIRE that Physician opt out of Medicare so that Medicare patients may be seen by the Practice pursuant to this private direct primary care contract. Neither Practice nor Physician make any representations regarding third party insurance reimbursement of fees paid under this Agreement. Patient shall retain full and complete responsibility for any such determination. If Patient is eligible for Medicare, or during the term of this Agreement becomes eligible for Medicare, then Patient will sign the agreement attached as Appendix 2, and incorporated by reference. This Agreement acknowledges your understanding that Physician has opted out of Medicare, and as a result, Medicare cannot be billed for reimbursement for any such services.

5. Insurance or Other Medical Coverage. Patient acknowledges and understands that this Agreement is not an insurance plan, and not a substitute for health insurance or other health plan coverage (such as membership in an HMO). It will not cover hospital services, or any services not personally provided by Practice, or its Physician. Patient acknowledges that Practice has advised that Patient obtain or keep in full force such health insurance policy(ies) or plans that will cover Patient for general health care costs. Patient acknowledges that THIS AGREEMENT IS **NOT** A CONTRACT THAT PROVIDES HEALTH INSURANCE, in isolation does NOT meet the insurance requirements of the Affordable Care Act, and is not intended to replace any existing or future health insurance or health plan coverage that Patient may carry.

This Agreement is for ongoing primary care, and Patient may need to visit the emergency room or urgent care from time to time. Physician will make every effort to be available via phone, email, other methods such as "after hours" appointments when appropriate, but Physician cannot guarantee 24/7 availability.

6. Disclaimer. This agreement does not provide health insurance coverage, including the minimal essential coverage required by applicable federal law. It provides only the services described herein. It is recommended that health care insurance be obtained to cover medical services not provided for under this direct primary care agreement.

7. Term. This Agreement will commence on the date it is signed by Patient and Physician below and will extend monthly thereafter. Notwithstanding the above, both Patient and Practice shall have the absolute and unconditional right to terminate the Agreement, without the showing of any cause for termination. Patient may terminate the agreement with twenty-four hours prior notice, but Practice shall give thirty days prior written notice to Patient and shall provide Patient with a list of other practices in the community in a manner consistent with local patient abandonment laws.

Reasons Practice may terminate the agreement with the Patient may include but are not limited to:

a.   Patient fails to pay applicable fees owed pursuant to Appendix 1 per this Agreement;
b.   Patient has performed an act that constitutes fraud;
c.   Patient repeatedly fails to adhere to the recommended treatment plan, especially regarding the use of controlled substances;
d.   Patient is abusive, or presents an emotional or physical danger to the staff or other patients;
e.   Practice discontinues operation; and
f.   Practice has a right to determine whom to accept as a Patient, just as a Patient has the right to choose his or her physician.
g.   Practice may also terminate a Patient without cause as long as the termination is handled appropriately (without violating patient abandonment laws).

8. Privacy & Communications. You acknowledge that communications with Physician using e-mail, facsimile, video chat, instant messaging, and cell phone are not guaranteed to be secure or confidential methods of communication. Practice will make an effort to secure all communications via passwords and other protective means and these will be discussed in an annually updated Health Insurance Portability and Accountability Act (HIPAA) "Risk Assessment." Practice will make an effort to promote the utilization of the most secure methods of communication, such as software platforms with data encryption, HIPAA familiarity, and a willingness to sign HIPAA Business Associate Agreements. This may mean that conversations over certain communication platforms are highlighted as preferable based on higher levels of data encryption, but many communication platforms, including email, may be made available to Patient. If Patient initiates a conversation in which Patient discloses "Protected Health Information (PHI)" on one or more of these communication platforms then Patient has authorized Practice to communicate with Patient regarding PHI in the same format.

9. Severability. If for any reason any provision of this agreement shall be deemed, by a court of competent jurisdiction, to be legally invalid or unenforceable in any jurisdiction to which it applies, the validity of the remainder of the Agreement shall not be affected, and that provision shall be deemed modified to the minimum extent necessary to make the provision consistent with applicable law and in its modified form, and that provision shall then be enforceable.

10. Reimbursement for Services if Agreement is Invalidated. If this Agreement is held to be invalid for any reason, and if Practice is therefore required to refund all or any portion of the monthly fees paid by Patient, Patient agrees to pay Practice an amount equal to the fair market value of Services actually rendered to Patient during the period of time for which the refunded fees were paid.

11. Assignment. This Agreement, and any rights Patient may have under it, may not be assigned or transferred by Patient.

12. Jurisdiction. This Agreement shall be governed and constructed under the laws of the State of Idaho and all disputes arising out of this Agreement shall be settled in the court of proper venue and jurisdiction for Practice address in Boise, Idaho.

13. Patient Understandings (initial each):

_____ This Agreement is for ongoing primary care and is not a medical insurance agreement.

_____ I do NOT have an emergent medical problem at this time.

_____ I am enrolling (myself and my family if applicable) in Practice voluntarily.

_____ I understand that I am enrolling in a membership-based practice that will bill me monthly.

_____ In the event of a medical emergency, I agree to call 911 first.

_____ I understand Physician at PRACTICE will make every effort to be available but may not always be
        able to see me on a same-day basis. I may be referred to an urgent care for same-day
        service.

_____ I do NOT expect the practice to file or fight any third party insurance claims on my behalf.

_____This Agreement does not meet the individual insurance requirement of the Affordable Care Act.

_____ This Agreement is non-transferable.

_____ I do NOT expect the practice to prescribe chronic controlled substances on my behalf.

(These include commonly abused opioid medications, benzodiazepines, and stimulants.)

_____ I understand failure to pay the membership fee will result in termination from Practice.

Patient Name

_____
_____Date _____

Patient (or Guardian) Signature

_____

Physician Name

_____

Physician Signature

_____
Date_____

APPENDIX 1: PRACTICE Periodic & Enrollment Fees and Services

This Agreement is for ongoing primary care. This Agreement is not health insurance.
Patient may need to use the care of specialists, ERs and/or urgent care centers that are outside of the scope of this Agreement. Each Physician within the Practice will make an appropriate determination about the scope of services offered by the Physician. Examples of conditions we treat, procedures we perform, and medications we prescribe are attached herein, listed on our website and are subject to change.

PRACTICE Fee Schedule:
Enrollment Fee - This is charged when Patient enrolls with Practice and is nonrefundable. If a patient discontinues membership and wishes to re-enroll in the practice we reserve the right to decline re-enrollment or to require a re-enrollment fee of $XXX.00.

Monthly Periodic Fee - This fee is for ongoing primary care services. We prefer that you schedule visits more than 24 hours in advance when possible. We do not provide walk-in urgent care services.

Enrollment fee is $ XX.00
Monthly periodic fee thereafter is:
- $XX.00 per month for patients 21 years of age and older,
- $XX.00 for patients 20 years of age and under OR $XX.00 for patients 20 years of age and under with an adult family member-patient of PRACTICE.

There is only one enrolment fee due per family members residing in the same household in a given calendar year.

Included Services:
Ongoing Primary Care and In-Office Procedures - There are no fees for office visits. Some procedures have a nominal additional fee to cover the cost of supplies. These are detailed below and are subject to change.

Laboratory Studies - will be charged according to the low negotiated direct price plus 10%.

Medications - will be ordered in the most cost effective manner possible for Patient. Medications dispensed in the office are made available to Patient at wholesale cost plus 10%.

Pathology - studies will be ordered in the most economical manner possible. Anticipated prices for these studies are listed below and on our website.

Surgery and Specialist Consults will be ordered in the most cost effective manner possible for Patient. We utilize a specialty consult service, "RubiconMD" when possible to save on Patient's on healthcare costs.

Vaccinations are NOT offered in our office at this time with the exception of flu shots, Tetanus, Tdap and special order immunizations. We will make an effort to help you obtain needed vaccinations at a low cost.

After-Hours Visits - There is no guarantee of after-hours availability. This agreement is for ongoing primary care, not emergency or urgent care. Physician will make reasonable efforts to see you and be available electronically as needed after hours if your Physician is available.

Acceptance of Patients - We reserve the right to accept or decline patients based upon our capability to appropriately handle the patient's needs. We may decline new patients pursuant to the guidelines proffered in Section 7 (Term), because Physician's panel of patients is full or because a Patient requires medical care not within Physician's scope of services.

Hospital Services and Obstetric Services are NOT a part of our membership. Physician may visit Patient if requested by Patient or a representative if Patient is hospitalized but Physician will not write orders.

Reference 4: Sample List of Services

	DPC Sample Services	
Services	Wellness Exams including Well Child & Sports Physicals	Included
	Same Day/Next Day Visits	Included
	Telemedicine visits (email, phone, video chat)	Included
Procedures	EKG	Included
	Ingrown Toenail removal	Included
	Skin Lesion Removal or destruction (warts, sun spots, etc)	Included
	Joint Injections (knee, shoulder, trochanter, epicondyle)	$20 (each)
	Skin Lesion Excision & Biopsy (does not include pathology fee)	$20
	Pathology fee for removed skin lesions	$65
	Laceration repairs	$20/stitches & $30/glue
	Pap Smears/ HPV Testing	$26 / $40
	Flu Shot	Included
	B12 Shot	$11
Complex Care	Diabetes Management	Included
	Hypertension Management	Included
	Hyperlipidemia (cholesterol) Management	Included

	Mental Health/Wellness	Included
	Hospital Follow-Up and/or Pre-Op Evaluations	Included
	Weight Management Planning	Included
Labs/Imaging	Urinalysis	Included
	Urine Pregnancy Test	Included
	Rapid Strep Testing and/or Rapid Flu Testing	Included
	Wellness Labs (cmet, cholesterol profile)	$10
	Thyroid Testing (TSH, free T4)	$10
	Diabetes labs (cmet, cholesterol, A1c)	$15
	All other labs	often <65% billed retail
	Chest Xray	$45
	Ultrasounds, CT scans, MRI studies	$125-$600
Medication Discounts	Discount Prescription Card and education about goodRx	Included
	In house drug dispensary with low cost generic drugs	Wholesale cost + 10%

Reference 5: Sample Medicare Beneficiary Addendum

Appendix 2: DPC clinic Name and Medicare Patient Understandings

This agreement is between DPC Clinic name and

Medicare Beneficiary: _____
Medicare ID:_____

Who resides at: _____

Patient is a Medicare Part B beneficiary ("Beneficiary") seeking services covered under Medicare Part B pursuant to Section 4507 of the Balanced Budget Act of 1997. Practice has informed Beneficiary or his/her legal representative that Dr. NAME at the Practice has opted out of the Medicare program.

Physician in Practice have not been excluded from participating in Medicare Part B under [1128] 1128, [1156] 1156, or [1892] 1892 of the Social Security Act.

Beneficiary or his/her legal representative agrees, understands and expressly acknowledges the following:

Initial
_____ Beneficiary or legal representative accepts full responsibility for payment of Physician's charge for all services furnished by Physician.
_____ Beneficiary or legal representative understands that Medicare limits do not apply to what the physician may charge for items or services furnished by the physician.

_____ Beneficiary or legal representative agrees not to submit a claim to Medicare or to ask Physician to submit a claim to Medicare.

_____ Beneficiary or legal representative understands that Medicare payment will not be made for any items or services furnished by Physician that would have otherwise been covered by Medicare if there was no private contract and a proper Medicare claim had been submitted.

_____ Beneficiary or legal representative enters into this contract with the knowledge that he/she has the right to obtain Medicare-covered items and services from Physician and practitioners who have not opted out of Medicare, and the beneficiary is not compelled to enter into private contracts that apply to other Medicare-covered services furnished by other Physician or practitioners who have not opted out.

_____ Beneficiary or legal representative understands that Medi-Gap plans do not, and that other supplemental plans may elect not to, make payments for items and services not paid for by Medicare.

_____ Beneficiary or legal representative acknowledges that the beneficiary is not currently in an emergency or urgent health care solution.

_____ Beneficiary or legal representative acknowledges that a copy of this contract has been made available to him/her.

Executed on:_____

By: Medicare Beneficiary or legal representative

And:_____

Dr. NAME on behalf of PRACTICE NAME, LLC

Reference 6: Dr. Vance Lassey's Tips for Navigating challenging hospital relationships in Direct Primary Care.
By Vance Lassey, MD

Direct Primary Care is a great example of disruptive innovation. Hospitals have very clear priorities, and regardless of what hospital administrators will say with their mouths, their actions say something different about their priorities, which can be summed up in one character: $. And they don't like that priority being disrupted.

As a Direct Primary Care physician (AKA "DPC Doc") you have left the world of corporate-speak, board meetings, wasted money, and consultants. You have embraced a common sense, high-quality, accessible, and affordable model of medical practice, one that is focused only on serving patients. But even though your priorities and those of the hospital differ, you still have something to offer each other, and achieving the best care of your patients requires you to work it out. Please note: being just fine with the status quo, hospitals care more about money than the best care for your patients, thus the responsibility of the "sell" is on you.

Although most DPC Docs don't offer it, I believe that the truly full-spectrum high-value continuity Family Medicine DPC package includes inpatient care. In our world of fragmented, low-continuity hospitalist care, you will have to negotiate to be able to offer your superior alternative.

Human nature tends to cause us to reject people who don't conform, and you will find that you (intentionally or unintentionally) are not well-received by hospital administrators. Typically, they *automatically*--almost reflexively--will be defensive and anxious when dealing with you from the first moment you interact. But, knowing this is coming, you can be 100% prepared for it, and ready to defuse the situation and find common and mutually beneficial ground and build a successful working relationship. When setting down with a hospital administrator to negotiate things like facility fees and even privileges, here are some keys to success:

Be confident, but kind. Hospital administrators are not comfortable dealing with doctors they don't "own". In the face of corporate pressure, to avoid confrontation, doctors traditionally give in. You absolutely can't give in, or compromise, and you have to be confident. If you're not naturally confident, *fake it, just like the first time you took up a scalpel and made an incision into another human being.* Be careful to avoid over-confidence, which will be interpreted as arrogance and will kill your negotiation. My personal key to pulling this off is to exude kindness and warmth, while being confident. Show that you care about them and the success and image of their hospital, and say that you want to be a leader on their winning team. (Your demeanor will demonstrate that you're a leader and a winner, and people are drawn to that.) Before presenting your requests and demands (the "whats and hows"), first state your "whys". Highlight your desire to provide excellent patient care, value, and service. Defuse defensiveness by reminding them of their own hospital's mission statement, and explain how your goals align with that.

Use logic to appeal to their need to turn a profit. I know this one seems counter-intuitive, because administrators usually don't make decisions based on logic or common sense. But they aren't traditional businessmen and women who produce a widget, know exactly what that costs to produce, and how much they need to sell it for to make the necessary profit. If they were, these interactions would be much easier. The hospital's "products" have a nebulous undefined value that is based more on "allowable charges" and RVU's and other confusing things. Steer them away from this kind of thinking and help them see how they'll make money, and how they'll make it quickly without paying business office people for 2 years of haggling to get paid by an insurance company. I recently sent this to a hospital's imaging department director:

> I'm going to quote you here: "Our prices are based on what we can get reimbursed from insurance companies." I understand that and I don't think there's anything wrong with your prices for insurance patients, after all, the hospital is going to have to pay people to submit claims, wade through Prior Auths, haggle for reimbursement, and will have to wait months to years to get paid. Using all those resources costs the hospital money.
>
> But cash patients burden you with none of those hassles. I would love nothing more than for the hospital to break out of the mindset of 3rd-party payors, and to think about cash patients like mine--patients with no insurance, high-deductible insurance, or Faith-Based Cost-Sharing plans who will be paying cash for your services. With our patients, insurance won't enter into the

equation, so don't think about "what insurance companies allow". Instead, think "How much money do we need to make on this procedure, and how badly do we need it?" Then develop a separate price list for cash-paying patients. They give you the money, you give them the x-Ray. End of transaction. They'd be saving you an awful lot of work, and giving them a significant discount is only logical, especially if you're competing with other imaging providers who have figured out how to make a profit while offering a deep discount to these patients.

Remember that you're the boss. In nature, there are lots of small animals that make themselves look big and scary in order to scare off bigger predators. Consider the peacock- a small bird, but with a huge fan of feathers covered in menacing-looking translucent "eyes." In the wild, they are preyed upon by big jungle cats like tigers. Some of their predators are stupid, and miss out on an easy meal because they totally fall for this "I look big and scary even though I'm a little bird" trick. In the business world, the boss is the one who pays the bills and payroll. When you admit a patient to the hospital, and they or their insurance company pay the hospital, the hospital employees get paid, including the CEO. By that definition then, as the doctor, you are the boss. You're the tiger at the top of the food chain. However, the administrators want you to think they're the boss, and they have lots of ways to threaten you. Don't be fooled by the threats and fakery of the peacock. When a smart and confident tiger keeps advancing on that bold peacock, eventually that bird will run. Hopefully this kind of thing is rarely necessary for you, but you have the moral high ground, and that's a winning place to be. If, without a logical reason, the administrator continues to block you from practicing the best care there is, then they've thrown up the feathers and advanced on you. So attack. A good way to do this is to be ready to go public with their refusal. There's nothing hospitals hate more than bad press. To a newspaper editor, a local doctor's story about a hospital's refusal to allow a doctor to care for her patient while trying to save the patient money is a juicy front page story or editorial. If you have to write the story, then write it (or write it in advance if you anticipate their lack of cooperation and have it up your sleeve). Show it to the administrator before taking it to the paper. Tell them it goes to the paper tomorrow. Then watch 'em fold up the scary feathers and cooperate.

You're blazing the trail so cut it wherever you want to go. In your area, you may be the only doctor trying to do private medicine and get hospital privileges, or the only doctor who wants to get cheap cash prices for vaginal delivery, or low cash prices on an MRI, or whatever it may be. If nobody's ever gone there before you, you're blazing the trail. There's no wrong way. Find creative solutions. Others may have cut a similar trail in their area, you can use their experience to guide you. But remember there's always more than one way home.

Know the stuff they don't know, and bring the proof with you. Have you ever called a store to ask if they have something in stock, and the person on the phone says sounds pretty inexperienced, and you can tell they don't know if they have it or not, but they suddenly answer "no" *way too quickly?* Your instinct immediately tells you that the employee doesn't know, and you're right.

You go to the store and there it is, right there on the shelf. The reason they lied and said no, is they have no vested interest in helping you find what you need. They get paid minimum wage and are happy for you not to come in at all. Hospital administrators operate in a similar fashion when asked about things they're ignorant about. Ironically, they SHOULD recognize their vested interest in you bringing them cash business, but they don't, because again, they're not traditional business people, they're focused on 3rd party payors. You may be asking them to allow you to do something new that they have no idea how it would work. So in their ignorance, they'll answer that it's illegal or not within Medicare guidelines etc. They're wrong. It's just way easier to deny your request than it is to look it up or figure it out.

Here's an example: I wanted to care for Medicare patients in the hospital, and order Medicare outpatient labs/X-rays there, even though I had opted out of Medicare. The hospital CEO said, over and over: "You can't do that, it's against Medicare rules." I knew it was possible, because I knew a DPC doc who was doing it at the time. The administrator just didn't know how to make it work, and was worried about the hospital not getting paid. It was easier for this individual to tell me "sorry that's against the rules." After weeks of reading boring Medicare guidelines, my wife finally found the necessary documentation, and I presented proof to the CEO that they would be paid for my work. And I was good to go. How much easier would it have been for me if I had that figured out before I ever asked, and brought the medicare documents with me? So use those of us who've already done this kind of homework (or if we haven't yet, do it yourself). Having done the work they were unable or unwilling to do, you'll have what you need to teach them, and now you have the intellectual and the moral high ground. You can't lose.

Transparently present their competition to them, and present it as their chance to win. This is pretty straightforward, and transparency helps everybody. If you have a competing facility offering you $175 Radiologist-read Mammograms, and you want them to give you them for $150, tell them you already have been offered $175 and you want them to beat it. You don't really have to tell them who's price it is, but if telling them gives you a strategic advantage (maybe it's a major competitor they're always trying to undercut) then go for it. Then if they give you the $150, go back to the first place and ask for $125. Get as many qualified entities as possible competing with each other, and continue until you've got the best possible price.

The End!

There's much much more to say. This book was the result
of a lot of trial and error and collaboration from 2014
through 2018. sparkMD is still open as of this publishing
and there is much more we have learned (and have done!)

Please remember, this is a guide, it is a how to for one
person (me) and is designed to help you.
Nothing sells better than authenticity.
Nothing grows a human better than work, compassion
and marching in the direction of your dreams.

So go out, be brave, be you, create something and don't
be afraid to change, to adjust, to reach out and to join an
amazing tribe of physicians.

Best to each of you!

Dr. Julie
President, DPCAlliance 2020-2022
Owner, sparkMD
Family Physician
Mom
Speaker
Hopeful Builder of People

Dr. Julie Gunther was raised in Boise, Idaho where she would have likely become a gypsy artist had she not been raised by an engineer and a microbiologist. After earning her undergraduate degree in Psychology at Harvard University, she worked in tech, did an about face, went back to school and enrolled in a non-degree conferring program at Vanderbilt University to completed her pre-med requirements and apply to medical school.

Dr. Gunther earned her Medical Doctorate (MD) from the University of Washington School of Medicine in 2005. She completed full-spectrum family medicine training in 2009 at Indiana University's Ball Memorial Hospital Family Medicine Residency in Muncie, Indiana.

Dr. Gunther has been interviewed about her practice, sparkMD by Forbes, NPR, Medical Economics, The Idaho Statesmen, PracticeLink and many more news outlets. She speaks on direct primary care and healthcare transformation for the American Academy of Family Physicians, the Doctors 4 Patient Care Foundation, the Hint Summitt and more. She is a founding member of the Direct Primary Care Alliance (DPCA), former Board Member of the Direct Primary Care Coalition and was instrumental in the passage of the State of Idaho's DPC legislation.

Dr. Gunther is a lover of all things art, particularly the work of Gustav Klimt. She has two tall, strong, independent daughters, two very needy Golden Retrievers and one infinitely patient, supportive and loving husband. She can be contacted at drg@sparkmd.com.

Made in the USA
Monee, IL
10 October 2023

44367594R00100